STUDY OF INTERACTION OF THE CYCLIN-DEPENDENT KINASE 5 WITH ITS ACTIVATOR, P25 AND WITH THE P25-DERIVED INHIBITOR, CIP

Antonio Cardone[1], R. Wayne Albers, Ram D. Sriram, Harish C. Pant

National Institute of Standards and Technology
Gaithersburg, MD 20899

National Institutes of Health
Bethesda, Maryland 20892

STUDY OF INTERACTION OF THE CYCLIN-DEPENDENT KINASE 5 WITH ITS ACTIVATOR, P25 AND WITH THE P25-DERIVED INHIBITOR, CIP

Antonio Cardone[1], R. Wayne Albers, Ram D. Sriram, Harish C. Pant

National Institute of Standards and Technology
Gaithersburg, MD 20899

National Institutes of Health
Bethesda, Maryland 20892

ABSTRACT

A high-affinity inhibitor protein called *CIP* , which can be produced by small truncations of *p35,* was earlier identified by Amin, Albers, and Pant. *P35* is one of the physiological activators of *cdk5*, a member of the cyclin-dependent kinase family. *P25* is an activator derived from the truncation of the physiological *cdk5* activator *p35* upon exposure to *Aβ* peptides, and it is known to be associated with the hyperphosphorylation of specific neuronal proteins. This typically occurs in the case of neurodegenerative diseases such as Alzheimer's. In this paper we study *in silico* the binding mechanism of *cdk5-p25* and *cdk5-CIP* complexes more in detail. This provides a better understanding of the inhibitory activity of the protein *CIP*. We use a geometry-based technique to verify the following hypothesis: *p25*'s truncation provides increased flexibility to *CIP*, and hence *CIP* is able to conform better to *cdk5* interface than *p25*. Therefore *CIP* is expected to bind to *cdk5* more easily than *p25* and prevent it from reaching its active conformation. Our *in silico* study is based on a geometry-based alignment algorithm. The algorithm is capable of efficiently aligning two protein conformations with respect to their interfaces, which are represented as point sets. The algorithm is based on biochemical criteria as well as geometrical ones. Our results indicate the validity of the flexibility hypothesis. They could be used, along with some observations we made on *cdk5* activation, as a basis for a set of very targeted and therefore more efficient molecular dynamics simulations.

Keywords: Cyclin-dependent kinase; neurodegenerative diseases; protein phosphorylation; computational geometry; feature-based shape similarity assessment; shape signature; point alignment algorithm.

1 INTRODUCTION

Cell functions are produced by chains of temporally interacting proteins that form complex networks. Major components of such networks are regulatory proteins that switch other components "on" or "off". Very commonly the regulator is a protein phosphokinase that transfers phosphate from ATP to a serine, threonine or tyrosine residue of the target protein. More than 500 protein phosphokinases are specified in the human genome. In their active states these

---

[1] Corresponding Author

1

proteins all have similar kinase domains, whereas their inactive conformations are quite variable: in many cases the active state is only formed after combination with an activator protein (i.e. the cyclin-dependent kinase family that regulates cell division). Other phosphokinases normally exist combined with an inhibitor protein that must be displaced by a regulatory event such as combination with a 'second messenger' molecule, such as cyclic AMP in the case of protein kinase A [Hus02]. Frequently kinases are subject to multiple regulatory mechanisms involving both conformational and covalent modifications [Hus02].

Cdk5, a member of the cyclin-dependent kinase family, differs from other members of this family in several respects: it has no known role in cell division; its activity is expressed primarily in mature (non-dividing) neurons; it is not activated by cyclins, but rather by two different physiological activators, *p35* and *p39*, which appear to have evolved independently of the cyclins. As the interface of *p35* and *p39* to the active conformation of *cdk5* is very similar to those of the other *cdk* family members, it is reasonable to assume that the kinase is activated by a mechanism similar to that proposed for other cyclin-dependent kinases: an active conformation of the comparatively flexible kinase molecule is attained upon binding it to a more rigid interface provided by activator protein [Jef95].

Interest in the above binding mechanism arose from a study designed to determine the minimal part of *p35* required for *cdk5* activation [Ami02]. In the course of this study it was observed that the 301 residues of *p35* when reduced to 154 (*p16* = Δ138-291) will fully activate recombinant *cdk5*. However, further small truncations produce a 126 residue, high-affinity inhibitor protein called *CIP* (*CIP* = Δ154-279) [Ami02]. Several neurodegenerative diseases are associated with hyperphosphorylation of specific neuronal proteins including, in the case of Alzheimer's (AD), the microtubule-associated protein tau which then aggregates within neurons to form neurofibrillary tangles. For instance, *cdk5* phosphorylates tau in correspondence of AD-specific phospho-epitopes when it associates with *p25*. *p25* is an activator derived from the truncation of the physiological *cdk5* activator *p35* upon exposure to *Aβ* peptides. Therefore hyperphosphorylation and formation of "neurofibrillary tangles" can be initiated by transfecting *p25* into neuronal cultures whereas co-transfection of *CIP* can prevent both [Zhe05].

Questions about the above-described binding mechanism might be addressed by directly simulating *cdk5-p25* and *cdk5-CIP* interactions. However, simulation of protein interactions is a computationally challenging task due to the complexity of protein structure and properties. On the other hand, advances in areas like computational geometry suggest that the above-described *cdk5-p25* and *cdk5-CIP* interactions might be initially addressed by studying their binding mechanism. In fact protein interactions need to be studied with reference to both their geometrical and their biochemical characteristics.

This paper is organized as follows. In the next section some of the most popular techniques that are available to model and simulate protein interactions are described. As geometrical shape characteristics and conformational transitions play a major role in protein interactions, dimensional shape similarity assessment techniques will also be covered in the literature survey. In Section 3 the problem in the current study is formally defined and the working hypotheses are stated. The working hypotheses focus on the geometrical aspects of the problem as well as on the protein biochemical characteristics. In Section 4 the geometry-based techniques to study *cdk5-p25* and *cdk5-CIP* interactions are described. In Section 5 the results of the study are presented and discussed. Finally, in Section 6 the conclusions are presented, along with our future plans.

2 LITERATURE SURVEY

Advances in bioinformatics in the past two decades have facilitated the structural identification of single protein three dimensional structures, obtained through X-ray diffraction and NMR (Nuclear Magnetic Resonance) techniques. However, only a fraction of the complexes consisting of more than one protein have been experimentally characterized. Therefore a number of computational techniques have been developed for characterizing protein structures and for simulating their interactions. Protein docking represents one of the most promising computational techniques to deal with this problem.

Protein docking can be defined as the prediction of the structure of a protein complex based on the independently solved structures of the components. The main challenge is to account for protein flexibility, which greatly increases the complexity of protein docking. Protein docking can be viewed as a process involving interaction and binding of two molecules where both geometric and chemical characteristics play a major role. Because of its nature docking is significantly more complex than an assembly problem of two rigid parts. For example the internal flexibility due to internal bond rotations needs to be considered for protein docking. Therefore a large number of variables are involved. Protein docking techniques can be classified based on the criteria used to predict the resulting protein complex. In this review we will cover purely geometric docking techniques and interaction energy-based docking techniques.

Purely geometric docking techniques [Nor99, Yue90] rely exclusively on protein geometric complementarity. Therefore, interaction energy and protein flexibility are accounted for indirectly. For instance, *soft docking techniques* account for protein internal flexibility by partially allowing overlapping of the interacting surfaces. Examples are BiGGER [Pal00] and FTDOCK [Gab97]. The latter relies on Fourier correlation theory. However, the accuracy of purely geometric techniques is not very high, as energetic terms and internal flexibility of proteins are not accounted for very accurately.

Energy-based docking techniques perform an explicit minimization of interaction energy, therefore accounting for internal flexibility in detail [Bur03, Kra99, Mor98, Ver03]. Modeling and minimizing the interaction energy function can be very complex, especially for large proteins. Several energy terms such as electrostatic, Van der Waals, solvation and hydrogen bond energies are required for computational accuracy. Each can have a very complex analytical form and may explicitly depend on the internal degrees of freedom of the proteins. For large proteins a very high number of degrees of freedom might be involved. Several attempts have been made to reduce the computational complexity of the problem, e.g., by limiting the flexibility of the proteins to only the surface side-chains. Other attempts have ignored the flexibility in certain surface areas based on biochemical criteria [Bet99, Con99]. Hence, in general energy-based techniques are more accurate than purely geometric ones, but they can be computationally intensive.

Among the energy-based docking techniques, the ICM technique is based on Internal Coordinate Mechanics (Figure 1) [Aba94a, Aba94b, Fer02]. It consists of rigid docking followed by flexible side-chain refinement based on energy minimization. The refinement is performed using a biased Monte Carlo flexible docking, where the internal parameter considered are torsion, phase and bond angles and lengths. The ICM Molsoft docking software uses the ICM technique. In the annual CAPRI (Critical Assessment of Protein Interactions) docking competition [Vaj04], ICM technique was shown to be one of the most accurate protein docking techniques. However, its efficiency can become very low if large proteins are involved (e.g. proteins with molecular weight higher than 10 kDa).

An alternative docking technique is based on the Lamarckian model of genetics applied to the minimum energy search [Hue07, Mor96, Mor98]. The Lamarckian genetic algorithm has been selected by the authors in after comparing its performance, on seven known dockings, to the following two search methods: Monte Carlo simulated annealing and a traditional genetic algorithm. The Lamarckian genetic algorithm can handle ligands with more degrees of freedom than the simulated annealing method and it proved to be the most efficient, reliable, and successful of the three algorithms. The docking software AutoDock is based on this technique [Hue07, Mor96, Mor98].

An additional energy-based docking technique employs a fast algorithm for energy minimization, based on an augmented Lagrange-multiplier method. In this case bond lengths, angles, and planar groups are constrained, while the potential energy related to torsions, hydrogen bonds, Van der Waals and electrostatic interactions is modeled by using elastic restraints. Then a local minimum of the total energy that satisfies the constraints is found by using the augmented Lagrange-multiplier method. The technique is user-friendly as it is possible to define user-specified springs, and its complexity grows linearly with the number of atoms involved. However, its performance is very good primarily on small proteins. This technique was used to build the software SCULPT, which is capable of modeling protein interactions in interactive computer graphics systems [Sur94].

Protein conformational changes are very important to protein function. For instance kinases are frequently subject to multiple regulatory mechanisms involving both conformational and covalent modifications. Protein docking techniques try to address the docking problem by accounting for conformational changes. However, accounting for conformational changes is computationally expensive because of the high number of variables involved. Therefore it is necessary to trade-off between efficiency and accuracy of the results, which is not an easy task. An alternative and in some cases more accurate method to study protein conformational changes is molecular dynamics (MD). MD techniques explicitly solve the well-known Newton equations of motion for all protein atoms and therefore they are able to predict protein conformational changes in detail. Most of the techniques that try to efficiently solve the problem are based on classical energy terms [And01, Ati01, Cas05, Hum96, Kal99, Lui00, Mou01]. However, in MD an acceptable accuracy of trajectories requires significantly short time steps. This makes MD simulations computationally expensive, especially for large protein complexes. In order to gain insight on protein dynamics without engaging in computationally expensive simulations, hybrid methods that couple MD simulations with collective motions derived from normal mode analysis (NMA) were developed [Tam00, Tam01]. In some cases the outcome provides insights about protein motions that go beyond the range of conventional molecular dynamics simulations. A potentially useful insight into the underlying principles governing protein dynamics and its relationship to protein functions can be derived from NMA techniques (see [Bah05] for a survey of NMA techniques).

An alternative to MD simulations uses the Lagrangian approach instead of the Newtonian approach, which is the primary technique used in the approaches described above. The Newtonian approach is fairly computationally expensive. On the other hand, the Lagrangian approach provides feasible atom conformations based on sets of constraints. The constraints are defined based on the biochemical characteristics of a protein complex. The software FIRST/FRODA is mainly based on the Lagrangian approach [Wel05]. It consists of two main modules: FIRST and FRODA. The FIRST module performs a rigidity analysis by balancing an atom's degrees of freedom with constraints based on biochemical criteria such as hydrogen bonds, covalent bonds and so on. In order to establish final atomic positions based on degrees of freedom and constraints, a pebble-game algorithm is used [Wel05]. The outcome is a rigid cluster decomposition of the protein (Figure 2). Then FRODA performs the protein dynamics simulation based on the rigid cluster decomposition. Interatomic potentials are represented by fictitious rigid bodies (referred to as *ghost templates*) that depict atoms' ideal positions according to the obtained constraints. So atoms are randomly displaced and then their positions are iteratively fitted to ghost templates [Wel05]. Due to the nature of the Lagrangian approach, FRODA is more efficient than traditional MD methods and it can be fairly accurate depending on the biochemical criteria used to define the constraints. However, the interaction energy is not explicitly minimized, as in MD simulations, and the outcome is not as accurate as in the MD case.

Protein geometric shape plays a major role in protein interactions. Often proteins with similar shapes have similar functions and/or interact similarly with their activators. Therefore, the study of proteins and their interactions might involve external shape similarity assessment. Over the last few years several algorithms for shape similarity assessment have been developed [Car03, Cam01, Iye05, Jay05]. As proteins are three dimensional entities, we will mainly focus on three dimensional shape similarity assessment algorithms. This problem can be efficiently solved by abstracting three dimensional shapes into shape signatures. Shape signatures are abstractions of the actual shape that completely characterize a three dimensional object. A shape signature can be represented by a matrix, a set of vectors or a graph. Therefore three dimensional similarity assessment involves computing the shape signatures and then comparing the shape signatures by a distance function. The distance function should ideally satisfy certain mathematical properties, such as identity, positivity and triangle inequality [Car03].

Three dimensional shape can be classified based on the shape signature that is used. The most common three dimensional shape similarity assessment techniques are based on spatial functions, shape histograms, section images, topological graphs and shape statistics [Car03]. In particular, feature-based techniques compute the shape signature of an object based on properties of the object's geometric features such as type, size, orientation and number. Once the features are extracted and their significant characteristics are determined based on the application, the three dimensional shapes are compared by using a distance function. Feature-based techniques discriminate the three dimensional models based on the features and their characteristics rather than the gross shape of the object. Feature interactions and multiple interpretations still pose significant challenges to successful extraction of features [Car04, Car06]. Some of these techniques appear to be promising for specific domains such as manufacturing cost estimation, while some others can be used as a filter to quickly prune dissimilar objects based on the shape similarity assessment criteria [Gup99, Kar05, Ram01].

Since feature-based similarity measures are defined using feature-based representations of objects, a three dimensional object is represented by a set of feature vectors. A distance function will provide the similarity measure between the two sets of feature vectors representing two objects. The distance function value depends on the relative positions and orientations of features. In particular, in order to compute the distance function, it is necessary to identify, for each feature belonging to one three dimensional object, the closest feature belonging to the other three dimensional object. The closest feature to a given feature is often referred to in literature as *closest neighbor*. Therefore, the distance value generally changes if a rigid body transformation is applied to one of the feature sets. From these considerations it can be inferred that feature-based shape similarity assessment involves finding the alignment between sets of feature vectors that minimizes the distance function. Such an alignment can be referred to as *optimal alignment*. This problem is directly related to point pattern alignment problems.

Considerable work has been done on the point pattern-alignment problem in several fields such as computer vision, pattern recognition, and computational geometry [Alt96, Hut90, Atk87, Alt88, Spr94, Alt88, Hef94, Mou99]. In the cases of two point sets with different cardinalities, the standard Hausdorff distance is used. This is based on the assumption that each point in one set has a close match in the other set [Che99, Hut92, Hut93a]. Alternative similarity measures have been used when such an assumption might not be valid. For instance the partial Hausdorff distance [Hut93b, Hut93c] allows some fraction of the points to be unmatched by minimizing the *kth* largest distance rather than the maximum distance. Other point pattern alignment techniques can be found in [Aga03a, Aga03b, Vel01]. In particular geometric hashing represents an important class of alignment techniques [Ira96, Wol97].

Based on the literature review we believe that the most accurate techniques for modeling and simulating protein interactions are computationally intense. On the other hand, based on recent advances in computational geometry, we think that it would be more convenient to initially study the geometrical characteristics of *cdk5-p25* and *cdk5-CIP* interactions rather than directly simulating them without having any insight. In the next section a more formal definition of the problem described in the introduction is given, and the working hypotheses are stated.

3 PROBLEM FORMULATION

One approach for studying our protein-protein binding mechanism would be to use MD simulations to compare *cdk5-p25* and *cdk5-CIP* interactions. However, as explained in the previous section, molecular dynamic simulations require hours of computer time to simulate nanoseconds of real time. Docking algorithms that employ approximations which permit mapping possible conformational trajectories independent of time are available [Fer02, Hue07]. Although some of these are able to predict the influence of small molecules on protein conformations, none appear adequate to predict conformational responses to protein-protein interactions. As a first step we have decided to analyze geometric aspects of this problem to decide if there are molecular dynamics criteria that may test our hypotheses by involving shorter timescale simulations.

Our work on this project is based on two main hypotheses: 1) the flexibility hypothesis and 2) the conservation hypothesis. The *flexibility hypothesis* is based on the following observations. Protein kinases are notable for assuming different conformations in response to interactions with different *cdk* regulatory proteins [Pav99]. In contrast, the *cdk* activator proteins, including cyclins and *p25*, interface with their kinases by means of a relatively compact, rigid and conserved 'cyclin box' consisting of 5 α-helices connected by short loops, which in the case of cyclin A does not significantly change its conformation upon complexing with *cdk2* (cyclin A structure can be found in [Bro95]). The N- and C-terminal residues removed from *p25* to produce *CIP* are helical in *p25* and they contact each other on the surface opposite the *cdk5/p25* interface. Their removal may relax structural constraints and introduce flexibility into *CIP* relative to *p25*. We suggest that increased flexibility may allow *CIP* to retain high affinity for the kinase interface while also producing inhibition by disorienting *cdk5* substrate binding at the kinase active site. Therefore the *flexibility hypothesis* shows that *p25* truncation that creates the inhibitory characteristics of *CIP* does so by increasing its flexibility relative to that of *p25*, such that the *cdk5/CIP* complex does not align the substrate protein or peptide with the catalytic site adequately to produce a significant rate of phosphorylation. This follows directly from the experiments described in [Ami02], which show that *CIP* inhibits *cdk5* activity with high affinity and competitively with *p16* or *p25* activation.

The *conservation hypothesis* is based on the following observations. *P35* is the principal physiological activator of *cdk5* expressed in neurons and consists of 307 residues. *P25* consists of *p35* residues 99-307 and combines with *cdk5* to elicit a higher rate of histone *H1* phosphorylation than *cdk5/p35*. *CIP* consists of *p35* residues 154-279. As this further truncation of *p25* at both N- and C-termini does not remove any residues that form the normal *cdk5-p25* interface (Figure 3), the *conservation hypothesis* asserts that the high affinity of *CIP* binding to the inhibitory interface with *cdk5* consists of some or all of the *cdk5-p25* interface residues on *cdk5*. It is important that all the interfacial residues need not be involved at every conformational state during the interactions that produce either activation or inhibition. In fact, looking at the known active and inactive conformations, it is clear that different parts of the *cdk5/p25* interface are subject to varying extents of conformational change. However, neither *p25* nor *CIP* components are expected to change as extensively as the *cdk5* component. A relatively small part of the interface is likely to interact first, and then, progressively, the rest of the interface will interact as *cdk5* conforms to more of the available interacting surface. In the case of its interaction with *CIP*, we expect that *cdk5* binding does not progress sufficiently to attain an active conformation. We refer to this progressive interaction as *zipper mechanism*.

We can now consider strategies for testing these hypotheses in more detail. One approach would be to obtain a set of geometrically and biochemically feasible *cdk5/p25* and *cdk5/CIP* intermediate conformations. Given these sets of conformations, the extent to which the two interface components, *cdk5* and *p25* or *cdk5* and *CIP*, remain similar can be compared. This, in turn, may be correlated with the conformation of the catalytic site.

Geometric affinity between protein conformations can be evaluated based on the conservation hypothesis: two proteins are geometrically affine if their interface is sufficiently close to the active conformation interface. If the resulting geometric affinities verify the flexibility hypothesis, then *CIP* conformations would be expected to adapt geometrically to more of the intermediate *cdk5* conformations than *p25*.

Based on recent advances in computational bioinformatics together with examination of the currently available structural data we believe that testing the flexibility hypothesis based on the conservation hypothesis is a feasible project from a computational perspective.

In the next section the problem formulated above is addressed. In particular, in Section 4.1 the method to obtain a set of geometrically and biochemically feasible *cdk5/p25* and *cdk5/CIP* intermediate conformations is described. Then in Section 4.2 the geometry-based algorithm to study the obtained protein geometric conformations is described after giving the necessary definitions.

4 METHODS

In this section our geometry-based technique to study *cdk5/p25* and *cdk5/CIP* intermediate conformations is presented. The technique consists of two following steps, which address the two tasks that were identified in the previous section. First, different *cdk5/p25* and *cdk5/CIP* conformations are obtained by using the software FIRST/FRODA. Then, the obtained *cdk5/p25* and *cdk5/CIP* conformations are analyzed by using our geometry-based algorithm. The algorithm outputs a distance value for each given protein complex. These distance values are used to compare the extent to which *cdk5/p25* and *cdk5/CIP* interfaces remain similar to their active conformations. Figure 4 gives an overview of our technique.

4.1 Obtaining protein conformations

The first task consists of obtaining sets of geometrically and biochemically feasible *cdk5/p25* and *p25/CIP* conformational trajectories. Given the protein sizes and the large conformational transitions involved, we chose to examine the conformational transitions using the FIRST/FRODA software. As explained above, FIRST/FRODA employs a constraint-based approach that efficiently explores the flexibility of proteins. It is not a purely geometrical approach, as the constraints are defined in relation to the conservation of covalent bond lengths and angles on existing hydrophobic and hydrogen bonds as well as on the avoidance of steric clashes. Therefore the internal flexibility of proteins that is evaluated by FIRST/FRODA employs both geometrical and chemical criteria.

A FIRST/FRODA simulation is typically run by using as starting conformation an initial, known protein (or protein complex) and as target conformation the desired final conformation of the protein (or complex). Given starting and target conformations, FIRST/FRODA will efficiently explore the flexibility of the protein complex and output feasible atom trajectories, if any. The obtained atom trajectories are such that the final protein (complex) conformation is reached within a user-defined approximation. Obviously there will be cases in which no feasible trajectories can be found.

Initially we tried to use FIRST/FRODA software to examine the behavior of the *cdk5/p25* complex directly. In fact our 'flexibility hypothesis' implies that *p25* is sufficiently rigid to resist most of the force of interaction without much distortion by *cdk5*, or at least more so than *CIP*. Therefore a *cdk5/p25* complex could be run through FIRST/FRODA using as target the *cdk5/p25* complex itself after replacing the *cdk5* active conformation with the inactive one.

However, a fundamental consequence of the 'flexibility hypothesis' is the fact that *cdk5* is likely to be activated by progressively combining with *p25* through the above-mentioned 'zipper' effect. Unfortunately this phenomenon could not be examined directly by using FIRST/FRODA software. In fact we preliminarily verified that if the correct force fields were applied between *cdk5* and *p25* in FIRST/FRODA, then as *cdk5* is forced by the program to go from the active to inactive direction, *cdk5* tends to detach from *p25* or from *CIP* when the 'normal' binding force is overcome by the imposed target force. Successive attempts to force the complex to interact resulted in a completely rigid *cdk5/p25* interface, which suggested to us that FIRST/FRODA is not a viable option for examining *cdk5/p25* complex directly. Therefore we decided to use FIRST/FRODA software to examine the conformational transitions of each protein individually using the procedures described in the following paragraphs.

The ideal data input for FIRST/FRODA consists of the initial and final coordinates of a protein. As mentioned in Section 3, an X-ray structure of the active complex, *cdk5/p25*, was obtained, but the inactive, unconstrained conformation of the *cdk5* molecule is yet to be synthesized. However, the cyclin-dependent kinases are a well-studied class. In particular *cdk2* kinase is a member with a primary sequence very similar to that of *cdk5*. It has been crystallized both as the unliganded, inactive form and also as an active complex, including one with cyclin A, Mg, ATP, and a peptide substrate (1qmz_Cdk2 file from [Bro95]). An unconstrained, inactive

8

cdk5 conformation can be obtained by homology with the unconstrained *cdk2* conformation (Figure 5).

At this stage it was possible to apply the FIRST/FRODA analysis using as the initial structure, the *p25*-constrained active *cdk5* conformation and, as the target, a homology structure of unliganded *cdk5*. The outcome of such a FIRST/FRODA analysis is a set of intermediate *cdk5* conformations that are geometrically and chemically feasible and are expected to predict the spatial trajectory of the inactivating conformational transition. In Figure 6 some of the generated conformations are shown. Note that the sampling frequency between the initial and the target conformations is a FIRST/FRODA user-defined parameter that determines the level of detail. Thus it is possible to estimate intervening conformations by using a pair of *cdk5* conformations determined by one run as initial and target conformations in a subsequent run of FIRST/FRODA.

The above-described procedure for obtaining *cdk5* conformations cannot be applied to *p25* or *CIP* based on currently available data since there are no closely homologous models. An alternative way of obtaining accurate *p25* and *CIP* conformations is employed based on the conservation hypothesis. The results are shown in Figure 7: on the left the active *cdk5/p25* complex is shown, and in particular its interface residues are marked; on the right a *cdk5* conformational change is shown with particular focus on an interface amino acid. Based on the conservation hypothesis we expect that *p25* and *CIP* interaction with any *cdk5* intermediate conformation will involve the same interface residues as the active conformation. Therefore, as shown in Figure 8, we represent the conformational changes of *cdk5* interface residues as vectors. Each vector represents a specific cdk5 residue displacement. Then, by using FIRST/FRODA, we bias *p25* and *CIP* interfaces to follow *cdk5* interface conformational changes. As shown in the figure, this is achieved by applying FIRST/FRODA to a given initial *p25* or *CIP* conformation by using the above-defined vectors as transformation biases. This way new *p25* and chemically feasible *CIP* conformations are obtained in compliance with the conservation hypothesis.

The above-described procedure can be more formally defined as follows:

For $i = 1$ to n-1, consider two given *cdk5* conformations $cdk5_i$ and $cdk5_{i+1}$ ($cdk5_0$ = active *cdk5* conformation, C_n = inactive *cdk5* conformation, n = number of obtained *cdk5* conformation)

1. For each *cdk5/p25* interface residue, obtain the set of directional vectors D_v representing each residue displacement from $cdk5_i$ to $cdk5_{i+1}$.

2. Apply FIRST/FRODA using the *i*-th *p25* conformation $p25_i$ ($p25_0$ = active *p25* conformation) as input without any target but with the directional vectors D_v as bias.

The same procedure is used for *CIP*, and it can be formalized likewise by just using the notation CIP_i for *CIP* *i*-th conformation.

As expected, based on the above observations *p25* and *CIP* were not able to adjust to all *cdk5* interface changes from active to inactive conformation. In fact after a few *cdk5* conformations the outcome of the above algorithm would not produce a feasible *p25* or *CIP* structure. As shown in Figure 9, at some point *p25* or *CIP* conformations resulting from the application of the above algorithm show unacceptable discontinuities in the backbone. Therefore

9

both *p25* and *CIP* are only able to follow *cdk5* conformational changes to a certain extent, as shown in Figure 10.

We know that FIRST/FRODA simulation accounts for significant biochemical characteristics such as covalent bond lengths and angles, existing hydrophobic and hydrogen bonds as well as steric clashes. Therefore several parameters need to be set to determine how the above-listed biochemical characteristics will affect the simulation. For a more detailed understanding of the parameters meaning and significance, refer to FIRST/FRODA User Guide, which can be found at [http://flexweb.asu.edu/software/first/]. Here we note that a trial and error procedure was used to fine-tune the parameter set.

Hence, after applying the above-descried procedures the following conformation sets are available:

- *cdk5$_i$* with $i = 0$ to n, where *cdk5$_o$* = *cdk5* active conformation and *cdk5$_n$* = *cdk5* inactive conformation.

- *p25$_i$* with $i = 0$ to m, where *p25$_o$* = *p25* conformation from *cdk5/p25* active complex and *p25$_m$* = *p25* last feasible conformation obtained.

- *CIP$_i$* with $i = 0$ to l, where *CIP$_o$* = *CIP* conformation from *cdk5/p25* active complex and *CIP$_l$* = *CIP* last feasible conformation obtained.

Observe that $n > l > m$, as shown in Figure 10. Also note that, for a given i, both *p25$_i$* and *CIP$_i$* conformations are obtained as explained above by referring to the interface conformational changes between *cdk5$_{i-1}$* and *cdk5$_i$*. Therefore any comparison between *p25* and *CIP* conformations should be performed between *p25$_i$* or *CIP$_j$* where $i = j$. Hence from now on we will refer to *p25$_i$*, *CIP$_j$* and *cdk5$_k$* conformations with $i = j = k$ as *corresponding conformations*.

Based on the obtained sets of geometrically and biochemically feasible conformations, it is possible to assess the geometric affinity of *p25* and *CIP* conformations with *cdk5*. This will allow us to verify whether the flexibility hypothesis holds.

4.2 Studying the geometric affinity of the obtained protein conformations

In this section the geometric affinity between corresponding conformations of *cdk5*, *p25* and *CIP* will be assessed based on the conservation hypothesis. We refer to the geometric affinity of two interacting protein conformations as the geometric similarity of their interaction with respect to the protein active conformation. The geometric affinity assessment will be used to compare *cdk5/p25* interaction to *cdk5/CIP* interaction in order to verify if the flexibility hypothesis holds.

The above-stated problem of geometric similarity assessment of protein interaction is addressed as follows, with the assumption that each protein conformation is considered rigid. First we define a unique geometric representation of protein interaction. Then, based on that, we define a protein interface *shape signature*. As mentioned above, shape signatures are defined as abstractions of actual shapes that completely characterize a three dimensional object. Then a distance function based on protein interface shape signatures is defined. The distance function yields the geometric affinity between corresponding conformations of *cdk5*, *p25* and *CIP* based on the conservation hypothesis. Finally we design an efficient algorithm to compute the previously defined distance function.

The next sections will describe the above stages in detail.

4.2.1 Unique geometric representation of protein interaction

Protein interaction can be seen as a complex network of single amino acid interactions that are arranged in space in such a way as to minimize interaction energy. In general both geometrical and biochemical aspects are important for interaction. Therefore protein interaction prediction and evaluation are complex tasks, as it is not only necessary to focus on geometric aspects but also to evaluate the biochemical characteristics of the amino acids involved.

In our case based on the conservation hypothesis our task is to evaluate how the interface structure varies with respect to that of the reference active conformation as the complex transits from the reference active conformation to an inactive state. This simplifies the task, as in analyzing protein interaction it is possible to reference the active conformation as a template. From this point on we will refer to the *cdk5/p25* interaction in this crystallized structure as *template interaction*.

The crystallized *cdk5/p25* complex is shown in Figure 11. A representation for *cdk5/p25* complex's interface information is needed. The criterion on which the representation is based is that atoms on amino acid residues from different peptide chains are interacting if their nearest approach is within 3.5 Å (see Figure 11). This numeric value is frequently employed for defining molecular interaction. By this criterion 22 amino acid pairs are identified. These 22 pairs will be our reference in this paper for representing the *cdk5/p25* complex's interface. Based on the conservation hypothesis we will evaluate interactions between the different conformations of *cdk5* and *p25* or *CIP*, providing a measure of how similarly the 22 pairs are interacting relative to their template interaction. Hence a unique geometric representation is needed to represent such interaction.

Based on the above observations we choose to represent protein interaction in this case at the amino acid level rather than at the protein surface level. In fact the template interaction can be exhaustively described by referring to the relative position and orientation of each amino acid pair.

Figure 12 focuses on a pair of interacting amino acids GLU42 and TRP190 from *cdk5/p25* crystal interface. We choose to represent a single amino acid in R^3 by referring to three atoms: α-carbon, backbone nitrogen and the atom that is closest to the interacting amino acid. In general we will refer to these as C, N and A, respectively. If the atom closest to the interacting amino acid is either the α-carbon, C or the backbone nitrogen, N, the carboxyl group oxygen is used instead (for the sake of brevity this case is not shown in the figure). We will refer to it as O. Therefore, as shown in the figure, each amino acid is represented by a triangle in R^3.

In order to uniquely represent the three dimensional position and orientation of an amino acid pair we need to define 6 independent parameters. In Figure 13 the chosen parameters are shown for the pair consisting of TRP190 from *cdk5* and GLU42 from *p25*. In order to formally define these parameters, we introduce the following definitions.

$$P_i = \{A_{1i}, A_{2i}\} \forall i = 1,...,22 \tag{1}$$

$$\vec{n}_{ji} = (\vec{C}_{ji} - \vec{A}_{ji}) \times (\vec{N}_{ji} - \vec{A}_{ji}) / \left\| (\vec{C}_{ji} - \vec{A}_{ji}) \times (\vec{N}_{ji} - \vec{A}_{ji}) \right\| \text{ for } j = 1, 2 \tag{2}$$

11

$$\pi_{ji} = \text{plane identified by } \vec{A}_{ji}, \vec{N}_{ji} \text{ and } \vec{C}_{ji} \text{ for } j = 1, 2 \tag{3}$$

In Equation (1) the set of amino acid pairs that identify the protein interface is defined, in Equation (2) the normal vector for amino acid A_{ji} is defined, where $\vec{C}_{ji}$, $\vec{A}_{ji}$ and $\vec{N}_{ji}$ are the position vectors of the above-defined C, A and N atoms from amino acid A_{ji} for $j = 1,2$.

Using equations (1), (2) and (3) it is now possible to formally define 6 parameters that uniquely identify the relative position and orientation of an amino acid pair P_i (see Figure 13). As it can be inferred from the figure, in order to define the 6 parameters three preliminary rigid transformations are applied to the amino acid pair P_i.

- Transformation *T1*: amino acid pair P_i is translated so that $\vec{A}_{1i}$ lies at the origin of the coordinate system.

- Transformation *T2*: amino acid pair P_i is rotated around the origin of the coordinate system so that $\vec{n}_{1i}$ is parallel to Z-axis.

- Transformation *T3*: amino acid pair P_i is rotated around Z-axis so that $\vec{C}_{1i}$ lies on X-axis.

The described transformations do not affect the relative position and orientation of the amino acids within pair P_i, as they are applied to both amino acids from the pair. The outcome of transformations *T1*, *T2* and *T3* is shown in Figure 13 where amino acid A_{1i} is TRP190 and amino acid A_{2i} is GLU42; amino acid A_{2i}'s position and orientation has changed according to the transformations. With respect to the new positions and orientations that have been obtained both for amino acid A_{1i} and for amino acid A_{2i}, the following set of parameters uniquely defines their relative orientation.

- α_i angle between $\vec{n}_{2i}$ projection onto coordinate plane XY and X axis
- β_i angle between $\vec{n}_{2i}$ and Z axis
- γ_i angle between $\pi_{2i} \cap \pi_{norm}$ and $\vec{C}_{2i} - \vec{A}_{2i}$ where π_{2i} is defined in (3) and π_{norm} is the plane identified by $\vec{n}_{1i}$ and $\vec{n}_{2i}$
- $\vec{d} = (d_{xi}, d_{yi}, d_{zi})$ relative position between $\vec{A}_{2i}$ and $\vec{A}_{1i}$.

Therefore, for each amino acid pair P_i, the relative position and orientation of amino acid A_{2i} with respect to amino acid A_{1i} is uniquely defined by a 6 component vector $(\alpha_i, \beta_i, \gamma_i, d_{xi}, d_{yi}, d_{zi})$. Observe that transformations *T1*, *T2* and *T3* are applied to the amino acids from pair P_i to simplify the parameters definition. However, this does not affect the generality of the definition. On the other hand, it is useful to formally define an algorithm to align two amino acids A_{2i} and A_{1i} based on a given parameter vector representing their desired relative position and orientation. In fact this algorithm will be extensively used later, and it is defined as follows.

Input:

- Amino acid pair P_i randomly positioned and oriented.
- Vector $\left(\alpha_i, \beta_i, \gamma_i, d_{xi}, d_{yi}, d_{zi}\right)$ representing the desired relative position and orientation for amino acid pair P_i.

Output:

- Amino acid pair P_i positioned and oriented according to vector $\left(\alpha_i, \beta_i, \gamma_i, d_{xi}, d_{yi}, d_{zi}\right)$.

Steps:

1. Translate both amino acid A_{2i} and A_{1i} from amino acid pair P_i such that both $\vec{C}_{1i}$ and $\vec{C}_{2i}$ are positioned at the origin of coordinate system (not exactly coincident to transformation *T1* above-mentioned since both $\vec{C}_{1i}$ and $\vec{C}_{2i}$ are moved).
2. Rotate both amino acid A_{2i} and A_{1i}, first around Z-axis and then around X-axis, such that $\vec{n}_{1i}$ is aligned to Z-axis (transformation *T2* above-mentioned).
3. Rotate both amino acid A_{2i} and A_{1i}, around Z-axis, such that $\vec{C}_{1i}$ lies on X-axis (transformation *T3* above-mentioned).
4. Rotate amino acid A_{2i}, first around Z-axis and then around X-axis, such that $\vec{n}_{2i}$ is aligned to Z-axis.
5. Rotate amino acid A_{2i} around Z-axis such that the angle between $\vec{C}_{2i} - \vec{A}_{2i}$ and X-axis ($\vec{C}_{2i}$ and $\vec{A}_{2i}$ both lay on XY coordinate plane) is γ_i.
6. Rotate amino acid A_{2i} around X-axis such that the angle between $\vec{n}_{2i}$ and Z-axis (they both lay on XZ coordinate plane) is β_i.
7. Rotate amino acid A_{2i} around Z-axis such that the angle between the projection of $\vec{n}_{2i}$ onto XY coordinate plane and X-axis is α_i.
8. Translate amino acid A_{2i} such that $\vec{A}_{2i} - \vec{A}_{1i} = \left(d_{xi}, d_{yi}, d_{zi}\right)$.
9. Apply to both amino acid A_{1i} and A_{2i} the following transformations in order to restore amino acid A_{1i} position and orientation:
   a. reverse of the rotation defined in Step 3;
   b. reverse of the rotation defined in Step 2;
   c. reverse of the translation defined in Step 1.

The various rotations mentioned in the previous algorithm can be obtained by using standard mathematical procedures to minimize a function of one independent variable [Bar94]. Figures 14 (a) to 14(h) show an instance of application of steps 1 to 8 of the above-defined algorithm.

The above-defined 6 component vector $\left(\alpha_i, \beta_i, \gamma_i, d_{xi}, d_{yi}, d_{zi}\right)$ uniquely defines the interaction between a single amino acid pair P_i. In general, referring to all the 22 amino acid pairs $P_i = \{A_{1i}, A_{2i}\} \forall i = 1,...,22$, we can define a set of vectors

$K_i = \left(\alpha_i, \beta_i, \gamma_i, d_{xi}, d_{yi}, d_{zi} \right) \forall i = 1,\ldots,22$, which uniquely defines the interaction between a given pair of proteins.

In the next section the shape signature for protein interfaces is defined based on their unique geometric representation.

4.2.2 Definition of the shape signature of protein interface

The shape signature for a three dimensional object can be expressed by a matrix, a set of vectors or a graph. Once the object shape signature is defined, it is possible to compare different objects by referring to their shape signatures. The geometrical details of the three dimensional shape that are included in the shape signature are closely related to the mathematical representation of the shape signature itself. Also, the efficiency of the method chosen to compare shape signatures will be affected by their mathematical representation. Therefore a shape signature should completely and efficiently characterize the three dimensional shape of the object. To efficiently define a shape signature it is important to realize that it need not necessarily account for all geometric characteristics, but just for the ones that are relevant for object representation.

A distance function will be used to evaluate the geometric affinity between corresponding conformations of *cdk5* and *p25* or *CIP*, guided by the conservation hypothesis. Thus, in accordance to the conservation hypothesis, the geometric affinity evaluation should be based on the interaction taking place in the crystal structure (file 1H4L.pdb from http://www.rcsb.org/pdb/home/home.do), which we defined earlier as the *template interaction*. In the previous section we identified 22 amino acid interacting pairs and defined a unique geometric representation at the atomic level. Based on this geometric representation, we decided to define a protein interface shape signature focusing on the closest atoms from each amino acid pair in the *template interaction*, as defined in the previous section for amino acid pair P_i by $\vec{A}_{ji}$ with $j = 1, 2$.

This choice transforms our protein interface geometric affinity assessment problem into a feature-based shape similarity assessment problem, where the features are the atom pairs, represented in general as attributed points in $\mathbb{R}^3$. Point attributes are transformation-independent characteristics of the atoms and/or amino acid whose location in space is represented by the coordinates of atom $\vec{A}_{ji}$. Feature-based shape similarity assessment is a problem that has been extensively addressed in the literature [Car03, Cam01, Iye05, Jay05]. Later it will be shown that our feature-based shape signature has useful mathematical properties. These mathematical properties allow us to define an efficient algorithm to compute a distance function that can be used to evaluate the geometric affinity between corresponding conformations of *cdk5*, *p25* and *CIP* based on the conservation hypothesis.

Let us define our shape signatures as follows: consider two interacting proteins, *cdk5ᵢ* and *p25ᵢ* or *CIPᵢ,*, and also an amino acid pairs list P_i that is based on the interacting amino acids from the template. The shape signature representing protein *cdk5ᵢ* interface is defined as a list of three dimensional points $\vec{A}_{1i}$ for $i = 1, 2, \ldots, 22$. Each point represents a particular amino acid from the protein conformation *cdk5ᵢ* interface, and any transformation-independent attribute can be attached to it. This also holds true for protein conformations, *p25ᵢ* or *CIPᵢ*: their shape signature is defined as a list of three dimensional points $\vec{A}_{2i}$ for $i = 1, 2, \ldots, 22$, and any transformation-independent attribute can be attached. These definitions reduce our problem to a three dimensional feature-based shape similarity assessment.

4.2.3 Definition of the distance function to evaluate protein geometric affinity

Our task is to evaluate the geometric affinity at the interface between a given protein pair based on the conservation hypothesis. As discussed above, the conservation hypothesis implies that the inhibitory interactions of *CIP* with *cdk5* mostly involve the same interfacial residue pairs as those that activate the *cdk5* kinase as a result of *p25* binding. We defined as the interactions of the 22 amino acid pairs at the interface of the crystallized complex of *cdk5* activated by *p25* the template interaction. Thus evaluating the geometric affinity between a given protein pair *cdk5_i* and *p25_i* or *CIP_i* involves assessing how close the interface between *cdk5_i* and *p25_i* or *CIP_i* is to the template interface, *cdk5_o*/*p25_o*. To accomplish this, we need the following definitions.

$$ K_i^0 = \left(\alpha_i^0, \beta_i^0, \gamma_i^0, d_{xi}^0, d_{yi}^0, d_{zi}^0 \right) \forall i = 1,...,22 \tag{4} $$

The vectors defined in Equation (4) are the unique geometric representations of the relative positions and orientations of the 22 amino acid pairs P_i^0 from the interface between *cdk5* active conformation, *cdk5_o*, and *p25* active conformation, *p25_o*.

$$ \mathbf{T_i^0} = \mathbf{T_i^0}\left(K_i^0, A_{1i} \right) \tag{5} $$

Equation (5) defines the transformation needed to align amino acid A_{2i} with respect to amino acid A_{1i} such that their relative positions and orientation are the same as in the template interaction. The transformation defined in Equation (5) is obtained from the transformations described in the algorithm ALIGN_RES_PAIR. In particular, using Equation (5) and referring to our shape signature, the following definition follows.

$$ \vec{A}_{2i}^t = \mathbf{T_i^0}(K_i^0, A_{1i})\vec{A}_{2i} \tag{6} $$

For a given *p25* or *CIP* conformation, $\vec{A}_{2i}^t$ is the atom $\vec{A}_{2i}$ location such that atom $\vec{A}_{2i}$ would be in the same relative position and orientation as in the active conformation with respect to atom $\vec{A}_{1i}$ from amino acid pair P_i. From now on we will refer to $\vec{A}_{2i}^t$ as *ideal location* of atom $\vec{A}_{2i}$ with respect to atom $\vec{A}_{1i}$. The expression *ideal location* is used because if, for two given corresponding protein conformations *cdk5_i* and *p25_i*, $\vec{A}_{2i} = \vec{A}_{2i}^t$ for $i = 1, 2,..., 22$, then *cdk5* and *p25* would interact exactly as they were interacting in the crystallized form. Based on the conservation hypothesis, that would mean that the interacting conformations, *cdk5_i* and *p25_i*, can interact with the highest possible geometric affinity.

From equations (4), (5) and (6) and from what was just stated we can infer that a technique to evaluate the geometric affinity between two given corresponding protein conformations is to compare how near the interface atoms $\vec{A}_{2i}$ from *p25* conformation *p25_i* (or *CIP* conformation *CIP_i*) are to their ideal locations, $\vec{A}_{2i}^t$. In other words, it is necessary to

15

evaluate the shape similarity between two three dimensional protein interfaces, namely between the *ideal interface* and the *actual interface*. This is a three dimensional feature-based shape similarity assessment problem, with the protein interface represented by sets of feature points. Based on the shape signature selected we will provide a general definition of the distance function to evaluate the geometric affinity between a given protein pair interface.

Observe that three dimensional objects in general and proteins in particular are represented in different coordinate systems. Therefore in order to assess similarity between two protein interfaces they need to be aligned such that the distance between the two corresponding sets of points is minimized. The aligning transformation that minimizes the distance between two sets of points is referred to as optimal feature alignment. Observe also that the point sets representing protein interfaces in general carry parameters other than their coordinates. In our case, point coordinates represent atom positions in the space, while other parameters could represent significant chemical characteristics such as atom type and residue type to which the atom belongs. We will refer to points carrying parameters other than their coordinates as *attributed points*.

Most of the available point alignment techniques mentioned in the literature survey involve identifying, for each point belonging to one set, the closest point from the other set in terms of the chosen distance measure (e.g. Euclidean distance). We will refer, given a point p from one set, to the closest point to p from the other set as *closest neighbor*. Therefore in general the distance function to compare two attributed point sets is defined as follows. Consider an attributed point p in R^3 represented by three transformation-dependent coordinates x_p, y_p and z_p and a transformation-invariant attribute w_p. For the sake of simplicity we define a single transformation-invariant attribute, which can be obtained as the combination of any number of transformation-invariant attributes without affecting the generality of the problem. The point sets A and B in R^3 can be compared using the following general distance function.

$$D(\mathbf{T}A, B) = \frac{\sum_{i=1}^{n} \min_{q \in B} d(\mathbf{T}p_i, q)}{n} \tag{7}$$

In Equation (7) $\mathbf{T}$ is the optimal alignment mentioned above and $d(\mathbf{T}p_i, q)$ could be defined as follows.

$$d(p, q) = \left(x_p - x_q\right)^2 + \left(y_p - y_q\right)^2 + \left(z_p - z_q\right)^2 + \left(w_p - w_q\right)^2 \tag{8}$$

Properties such as positivity, identity, symmetry and triangle inequality may or may not be satisfied for a given distance function. In this case positivity and identity properties are satisfied. The distance function defined in Equation (7) does not satisfy triangle inequality because it consists of a summation of quadratic terms. However, it is easy to differentiate, which is a highly desirable property.

The distance function $D(\mathbf{T}A, B)$ defined in Equation (7) changes with the aligning transformation $\mathbf{T}$. Hence, as mentioned above, it is necessary to evaluate the optimal alignment $\mathbf{T}$ that minimizes the distance function. This is, in general, a hard problem, as 6 degrees of freedom (DOFs) are involved in aligning two sets of points that are rigidly moving in R^3. Furthermore, as can be noticed by Equation (7), in order to evaluate $D(\mathbf{T}A, B)$ it is necessary to know the closest point q from set B for each point p_i from set A based on distance function $d(\mathbf{T}p_i,q)$. This makes the problem even harder. In fact standard minimization techniques cannot be used as, in general, the closest point q from set B to a given point p_i from set A changes as transformation $\mathbf{T}$ is applied to set A [Car06]. In particular, among the feasible values of transformation $\mathbf{T}$ there will be some specific values in correspondence of which the closest point q from set B to a given point p_i from set A will change [Car06]. For a 2 DOF instance that is simpler to visualize, it can be seen that the transformation space for a given point p_i of set A is divided into a set of subspaces such that its closest neighbor does not change within them (see Figure 15). Therefore $D(\mathbf{T}A,B)$ should be minimized within each subspace, and then the minimum value over all subspaces should be computed [Car06]. In general this is a computationally complex problem to address. However, in our case the conservation hypothesis significantly simplifies the problem from a computational perspective. In fact the distance function that is needed to evaluate the geometric affinity between protein interfaces is slightly different from the one defined in Equation (7). Our distance function is formally defined in the following paragraphs.

Let us consider the following protein conformations: cdk5 k-th conformation $cdk5_k$, p25 k-th conformation $p25_k$ and CIP k-th conformation CIP_k. For the k-th conformations, equations (1), (2) and (3) can be written as follows.

$$P_i^k = \left\{ A_{1i}^k, A_{2i}^k \right\} \forall i = 1,...,22 \tag{9}$$

$$\vec{n}_{ji}^k = \left(\vec{C}_{ji}^k - \vec{A}_{ji}^k \right) \times \left(\vec{N}_{ji}^k - \vec{A}_{ji}^k \right) / \left\| \left(\vec{C}_{ji}^k - \vec{A}_{ji}^k \right) \times \left(\vec{N}_{ji}^k - \vec{A}_{ji}^k \right) \right\| \text{ for } j = 1, 2 \tag{10}$$

In equations (9) and (10) the set of amino acid pairs representing the interface and the normal vector for amino acid A_{1i}^k are defined, where $\vec{C}_{ji}^k$, $\vec{A}_{ji}^k$ and $\vec{N}_{ji}^k$ are the position vectors of the above-defined C, A and N atoms for amino acid A_{ji}^k for $j = 1,2$. Other definitions referring to amino acid pairs can be changed accordingly. In particular the definitions from equations (5) and (6) can be modified as follows for the k-th conformations.

$$\mathbf{T}_{\mathbf{i}}^{\mathbf{0k}} = \mathbf{T}_{\mathbf{i}}^{\mathbf{0k}} \left(\mathrm{K}_i^0, A_{1i}^k \right) \tag{11}$$

$$\vec{A}_{2i}^{tk} = \mathbf{T}_{\mathbf{i}}^{\mathbf{0k}} (\mathrm{K}_i^0, A_{1i}^k) \vec{A}_{2i}^k \tag{12}$$

Finally, let us define the amino acid sets representing the shape signature of actual and ideal interface as $A^k = \left\{ \vec{A}_{2i}^k \right\} \forall i = 1,...,22$ and $B^k = \left\{ \vec{A}_{2i}^{tk} \right\} \forall i = 1,...,22$. Now it is possible to rewrite the distance function defined in Equation (7) as follows.

$$D^k(\mathbf{T}A^k, B^k) = \frac{\sum_{i=1}^{22} d(\mathbf{T}\vec{A}_{2i}^k, \vec{A}_{2i}^{tk})}{22} \tag{13}$$

In Equation (13), $d(\mathbf{T}\vec{A}_{2i}^k, \vec{A}_{2i}^{tk})$ is defined as follows.

$$d(p,q) = (x_a - x_b)^2 + (y_a - y_b)^2 + (z_a - z_b)^2 \qquad (14)$$

where $\mathbf{T}\vec{A}_{2i}^{k} = (x_a, y_a, z_a)$ and $\vec{A}_{2i}^{tk} = (x_b, y_b, z_b)$. Please note that the distance function defined in Equation (13) differs in two ways with respect to the general one defined in Equation (7). One difference is that as we are using the conservation hypothesis the distance function does not require identifying the closest neighbors anymore. In fact our task is to align as closely as possible the actual protein interface to the ideal one. Therefore the amino acid pairs that interact (i.e. that are closer to each other) are already known. This makes the distance function easier to compute. Furthermore, referring to Equation (14), another difference is that point attributes are not explicitly accounted for. This is because the biochemical characteristics of the interface amino acids are incorporated in the conservation hypothesis, as both the unique geometric representation and the ideal interface are based on amino acid biochemical properties. Therefore point attributes, which represent atom biochemical characteristics, are implicitly accounted for in the very definition of point sets.

At this stage the distance function $D^k(\mathbf{T}A^k, B^k)$ defined in Equation (13) can be computed after finding the alignment transformation $\mathbf{T}$. The next section will describe an algorithm to do this.

4.2.4 Alignment algorithm to evaluate distance function yielding protein geometric affinity

In this section an alignment algorithm to compute the distance function defined in Equation (13) is presented. The resulting distance value will yield the geometric affinity between *cdk5* and *p25* or *CIP k*-th conformation. Observe that, based on the definitions and related observations in the previous section, this is a computationally feasible task because of the characteristics of the biochemical problem we are addressing. In fact we intend to evaluate the geometric affinity between pairs of corresponding protein conformations based on the conservation hypothesis. This means that we need to compare the previously defined actual and ideal interfaces of *p25* or *CIP k*-th conformation. Therefore the mathematical form of the distance function and the related alignment problem are significantly simplified.

We mentioned that aligning two sets of attributed applied vectors in R^3 is a six degree of freedom problem. However, the protein interface characteristics can be used to discriminate among the possible alignments and therefore to decrease the computational complexity of the problem. Based on the conservation hypothesis and on the zipper-mechanism described in Section 3, we expect at least one interface amino acid pair to interact very similarly to the template interaction. As our approach involves the comparison between the actual and ideal interface of the same protein (either *p25* or *CIP*), the optimal alignment should have at least one amino acid pair from the actual interface very closely positioned with respect to the corresponding pair from the ideal interface. By applying the described preliminary alignment to a given amino acid pair five degrees of freedom are constrained. After the alignment the only degree of freedom left is a rotation around the axis identified by the aligned amino acid pair (refer to Figure 16). As it will be explained more in detail in the algorithm steps described below, each amino acid pair is aligned in two different ways, each corresponding to one amino acid from the pair. Therefore the total number of alignments in the case of 22 pairs is equal to the permutations P(22,2) = 462.

In order to evaluate the distance function defined in Equation (13), it is necessary to perform $P(22,2) = 462$ preliminary amino acid pair alignments and for each of them solve the corresponding one degree of freedom alignment problem. This is a computationally feasible problem because we are able to analytically minimize the distance function from Equation (13). The minimization is performed with respect to the one degree of freedom rotation shown in Figure 16. As observed above, both the distance function defined in Equation (7) and the one defined in Equation (14) do not satisfy the triangle inequality because they consist of a summation of quadratic terms. However the derivative is such that the summation of quadratic terms can be analytically minimized with respect to the one degree of freedom rotation. The algorithm that is used to compute the distance function defined in Equation (13) is presented as follows.

Algorithm: COMPUTEKTHDISTANCEFUNCTION

Input:

- $A^k = \left\{ \vec{A}_{2i}^k \right\}_{i \in [1,22]} = \left(x_i^k, y_i^k, z_i^k \right) \forall i \in [1,22]$, which are the actual atom locations from corresponding amino acid pairs P_i defined above for k-th protein conformations.

- $B^k = \left\{ \vec{A}_{2i}^{tk} \right\}_{i \in [1,22]} = \left(x_i^{tk}, y_i^{tk}, z_i^{tk} \right) \forall i \in [1,22]$ set of the ideal atom locations from corresponding amino acid pairs P_i defined above for k-th protein conformations.

Output:

- Value $D_{\min}^k$ of the distance function $D^k(\mathbf{T}^k A^k, B^k)$ defined in Equation (13) corresponding to aligning transformation $\mathbf{T}^k$ for k-th protein conformations.

Steps:

1. For $i = 1$ to 22

    For $j = 1$ to 22, $j \neq i$

       i. Apply the translation $\mathbf{Tr}_i$ to set A^k such that $\vec{A}_{2i}^k = \vec{A}_{2i}^{tk}$.

       ii. If $\vec{A}_{2i}^{tk} \neq \vec{A}_{2j}^{tk}$

           a. Apply the rotation $\mathbf{R}_{ij}$ around pivot point $\vec{A}_{2i}^k = \vec{A}_{2i}^{tk}$ to set A^k such that $\vec{A}_{2j}^k$ is located as close as possible to $\vec{A}_{2j}^{tk}$, which means that $\vec{A}_{2j}^k$ lies on the line through $\vec{A}_{2i}^k = \vec{A}_{2i}^{tk}$ and $\vec{A}_{2j}^{tk}$ (see Figure 17).

           b. Define the rotation axis r as the line passing through atom locations $\vec{A}_{2i}^k$ and $\vec{A}_{2j}^k$.

       Else

           c. Define the rotation axis r based on the locations of the atoms $\vec{A}_{1i}^k$ and $\vec{A}_{1j}^k$ above defined.

           d. Apply the rotation $\mathbf{R}_{ij}$ around pivot point $\vec{A}_{2i}^k = \vec{A}_{2i}^{tk}$ to set A^k such that $\vec{A}_{2j}^k$ lies on the line through $\vec{A}_{2i}^k = \vec{A}_{2i}^{tk}$ and parallel to rotation axis r (see Figure 18).

---

iii. Compute the rotation ϑ_{ij} and corresponding rotation matrix $\mathbf{R}(\vartheta_{ij})$ around axis r defined in Step 1.ii that minimizes the distance function $D^k(\mathbf{Tr_i R_{ij} R}(\vartheta)A^k, B^k)$ (see Figure 19).

iv. Compute the minimum distance $D^k_{ij} = D^k(\mathbf{Tr_i R_{ij} R}(\vartheta_{ij})A^k, B^k)$.

2. Identify the minimum distance value over all alignments from Step 1: $D^k_{min} = \min\limits_{ij} D^k_{ij} = D^k_{\bar{i}\bar{j}}$. The corresponding aligning transformation is $T^k = \mathbf{Tr_{\bar{i}} R_{\bar{i}\bar{j}} R}(\vartheta_{\bar{i}\bar{j}})$.

Observe that in Step 1.ii of the algorithm COMPUTEKTHDISTANCEFUNCTION the cases in which $\vec{A}^{tk}_{2i} = \vec{A}^{tk}_{2j}$ are specifically addressed. Such cases are possible because both $\vec{A}^{tk}_{2i}$ and $\vec{A}^{tk}_{2j}$ are ideal (i.e. not actual but theoretical) atom locations, and therefore they might be coincident. Hence no rotation axis r could be defined based on them. This is the reason why steps 1.ii.c and 1.ii.d define the rotation axis r based on atoms $\vec{A}^k_{1i}$ and $\vec{A}^k_{1j}$ from amino acids A_{1i} and A_{1j}. Amino acids A_{1i} and A_{1j} can be used because they are distinct amino acids belonging to *cdk5* real interface. Therefore we are guaranteed that $\vec{A}^k_{1i} \neq \vec{A}^k_{1j}$, otherwise two distinct atoms would hold the same spatial position, which is physically impossible.

The rotation ϑ_{ij} around axis r that minimizes the distance function $D^k(\mathbf{Tr_i R_{ij} R}(\vartheta)A^k, B^k)$ from Step 1.iii of algorithm COMPUTEKTHDISTANCEFUNCTION is formally defined in the next paragraphs. As shown in Figure 19 we can assume, without loss of generality, that axis r has been previously aligned to Z-axis.

The quantities d^k_g and ϑ^g_0 in Figure 19 are defined as follows.

$$\begin{cases} d^k_g = \text{constant distance of point } \vec{A}^k_{2g} \text{ from rotation axis corresponding to Z-axis} \\ \vartheta^g_0 = \text{initial angle between the projection of } \vec{A}^k_{2g} \text{ onto coordinate plane XY and X-axis} \end{cases}$$ (15)

Now, the distance function from Equation (13) can be written as follows.

$$D^k(\mathbf{R}(\vartheta)A^k, B^k) = \frac{\sum\limits_{g=1}^{22} d(\mathbf{R}(\vartheta)\vec{A}^k_{2g}, \vec{A}^{tk}_{2g})}{22}$$ (16)

In equation (16) ϑ represents the one degree of freedom rotation around the rotation axis r corresponding to Z-axis. Equation (14) also gets modified as follows, based on the definitions from Equations (15).

$$d(\mathbf{R}(\vartheta)\vec{A}^k_{2g}, \vec{A}^{tk}_{2g}) = \left(d^k_g \cos(\vartheta + \vartheta^i_o) - x^{tk}_g\right)^2 + \left(d^k_g \sin(\vartheta + \vartheta^g_o) - y^{tk}_g\right)^2 + \left(z^k_g - z^{tk}_g\right)^2$$ (17)

20

In Equation (17) $(x_g^{tk}, y_g^{tk}, z_g^{tk})$ are the coordinates of $\vec{A}_{2g}^{tk}$. In order to find the minimum value of the distance function from Equation (16) the following condition needs to hold.

$$\frac{\partial D^k(\mathbf{R}(\vartheta)A^k, B^k)}{\partial \vartheta} = 0 \tag{18}$$

The values of the rotation ϑ that satisfies Equation (18) is computed as follows.

$$\vartheta = \tan^{-1}\left(\frac{\sum_{g=1}^{22} d_g^k N_g^k}{\sum_{g=1}^{22} d_g^k M_g^k}\right) \tag{19}$$

In Equation (19) the quantities N_g^k and M_g^k are defined as follows.

$$\begin{cases} N_g^k = x_g^{tk}\cos(\vartheta_o^g) + y_g^{tk}\sin(\vartheta_o^g) \\ M_g^k = x_g^{tk}\sin(\vartheta_o^g) - y_g^{tk}\cos(\vartheta_o^g) \end{cases} \tag{20}$$

A given ϑ value resulting from Eq. (19) represents a local or global minimum only if the corresponding second derivative value from Equation (18) is positive. Therefore we select the ϑ value that minimizes the distance function from Equation (16) based on the sign of the second derivative.

Equation (19) yields the value ϑ corresponding to the best possible aligning rotation between the two amino acid sets A^k and B^k defined above. The aligning rotation is performed around a fixed axis through two amino acids $\vec{A}_{2i}^k$ and $\vec{A}_{2j}^k$ from set A^k. The two amino acids $\vec{A}_{2i}^k$ and $\vec{A}_{2j}^k$ defining the fixed rotation axis are aligned to their respective ideal locations. Therefore, for each amino acid alignment pair, it is possible to analytically obtain the optimal aligning rotation. Hence, as observed above, the algorithm COMPUTEKTHDISTANCEFUNCTION performs all possible amino acid pair alignments and for each of them optimally solves the corresponding one degree of freedom alignment problem. Therefore the resulting minimum distance value $D_{\min}^k = \min_{i,j} D_{ij}^k = D_{\bar{i}\bar{j}}^k$, whose corresponding aligning transformations is $T^k = \mathbf{Tr}_{\bar{i}}\mathbf{R}_{\bar{i}\bar{j}}\mathbf{R}(\vartheta_{\bar{i}\bar{j}})$, gives an accurate measure of the geometric similarity between the two feature sets A^k and B^k. Feature set A^k represents the amino acids belonging to the actual interface of a given protein conformation. Feature set B^k represents the ideal position, based on the conservation hypothesis, of the amino acids belonging to the interface of a given protein conformation.

The algorithm COMPUTEKTHDISTANCEFUNCTION for computing the distance function defined in Equation (13) is presented in this section. The resulting distance value gives an accurate measure of the geometric affinity between the interfaces of corresponding protein conformations based on their known active conformations. The algorithm is based on a discrete representation of protein interfaces as attributed point sets, where each point represents an amino acid belonging to the protein interface. This allows for the characteristics of protein interface at amino acid and atomic level to be considered. Furthermore, by using the known active protein conformations as reference, the point alignment problem corresponding to the geometric affinity assessment is significantly simplified. This simplification is due to the use of previously studied amino acid interactions from the active protein complex. This increases the efficiency of the feature point set alignment algorithm, maintaining a good accuracy level.

In the next section the algorithm COMPUTEKTHDISTANCEFUNCTION will be used to compare the geometric affinity of the proteins $p25$ and CIP to the cyclin-dependent kinase $cdk5$. In particular, Section 5.1 provides details about how our algorithm is applied to the available protein conformations. Then in Section 5.2 the results are presented and finally in Section 5.3 they are discussed.

5 RESULTS AND DISCUSSION

5.1 Description of algorithm application

A software system has been implemented based on the above-described COMPUTEKTHDISTANCEFUNCTION algorithm in Matlab on a Windows platform. As described in Section 4.1 $cdk5$, $p25$ and CIP conformations have been obtained using the software FIRST/FRODA. $Cdk5$ conformations have been obtained by using the crystallized $cdk5$ active conformation as initial conformation and the $cdk2$-like homology inactive conformation as target conformation. FIRST/FRODA sampling frequency has been set to obtain a total of $n \approx 14300$ conformations. Then $p25$ and CIP conformations have been obtained by biasing their interface amino acids to follow $cdk5$ conformational changes in compliance with the conservation hypothesis by using FIRST/FRODA. Among the obtained $p25$ and CIP conformations corresponding to the $n \approx 14300$ $cdk5$ conformations, only about 3000 conformations, starting from the crystallized one, are geometrically and chemically feasible. In fact the majority of the obtained conformations show breaks in the backbone. This means that $p25$ or CIP were not able to follow $cdk5$ conformational changes all the way to conformation of unliganded $cdk5$, in compliance with the conservation hypothesis. This was not surprising as $cdk5$ is expected to be more flexible than $p25$ and CIP. So finally only l CIP conformations and m $p25$ conformations are considered, with $l > m$ and both l and $m \approx 3000$.

Therefore, referring to these available data, the following inputs are given to the system.

- Files in pdb format [www.rcsb.org/pdb] representing the $p25$ feasible conformations obtained as described in Section 4.1. The $p25$ conformations were defined as $p25_i$ for each $i = 0$ to m, where $p25_o$ is the active conformation and $p25_m$ is last feasible conformation available (refer to Section 4.1 for details).

- Files in pdb format representing some of the feasible CIP conformations obtained as described in Section 4.1. The CIP conformations were defined as CIP_i for each $i = 0$ to l, where CIP_o is the active conformation and CIP_l is the last feasible conformation available. As $l > m$, we will focus only on the conformations CIP_i for each $i = 1$ to m (refer to Section 4.1 for details).

22

- Files in pdb format representing some of the *cdk5* conformations obtained as described in Section 4.1. The *cdk5* conformations were defined as $cdk5_i$ for each $i = 0$ to n, where $cdk5_o$ is the active conformation and $cdk5_n$ is the inactive conformation. As $n > m$, we will focus only on the conformations $cdk5_i$ for each $i = 1$ to m (refer to Section 4.1 for details).

- List of 22 amino acid pairs from active *cdk5/p25* complex interface.

- Vectors $K_i^0 = \left(\alpha_i^0, \beta_i^0, \gamma_i^0, d_{xi}^0, d_{yi}^0, d_{zi}^0 \right) \forall i = 1,...,22$ representing the relative position and orientation of the 22 interface amino acid pairs P_i^0 between *cdk5* active conformation $cdk5_o$ and the corresponding *p25/CIP* conformation $p25_o/CIP_o$.

The alignment is performed using the COMPUTEKTHDISTANCEFUNCTION algorithm and it yields a measure of the geometric affinity between corresponding *cdk5*, *p25* and *CIP* conformations ($cdk5_i$, $p25_i$ and CIP_i for the same i). In Figure 20 a schematic view of the software system that has been implemented is shown. Then, in Figure 21 an example of the application of COMPUTEKTHDISTANCEFUNCTION algorithm to a pair of protein conformations is also shown. The geometric affinity measure is based on the distance function described in Section 4.2.3. Therefore *p25* and *CIP* corresponding conformations can be compared based on this distance function: smaller distance values correspond to higher geometric affinities.

Our software data structure is consistent with pdb file format, which is one of the most commonly used file formats for representing proteins [www.rcsb.org/pdb]. It is also compatible with virtually any protein representation and modification software, such as SwissPro, VMD, NAMD.

COMPUTEKTHDISTANCEFUNCTION algorithm is applied to selected sets of corresponding *p25*, *CIP* and *cdk5* conformations to evaluate their geometric affinity based on the conservation hypothesis. For instance, two given *p25* and *cdk5* conformations are geometrically affine if their interface is very close to the active conformation interface. Our algorithm application will determine if the geometric affinities verify the flexibility hypothesis, i.e. if *cdk5/CIP* conformations remain geometrically affine over a greater range of conformations than *cdk5/p25*. Before applying the COMPUTEKTHDISTANCEFUNCTION algorithm to a given protein pair, note that the distance function $D^k(\mathbf{T}^k A^k, B^k)$ defined in Equation (13) is significant only if sets A^k and B^k actually represent protein interface amino acids. In some cases, two protein conformations could be such that the two proteins do not interact anymore and, hence, no protein interface is defined. A geometric criterion is needed to identify such cases.

Observe that sets A^k and B^k are defined based on the interface of the active *cdk5/p25* complex. Hence, they actually represent protein interface amino acids for the active conformation. Intuitively, A^k and B^k are very likely to represent actual protein interface amino acids for protein conformations other than the active one if such conformations are very close geometrically to *cdk5/p25* and *cdk5/CIP* active conformations. However, if larger protein conformational changes occur with respect to *cdk5/p25* and *cdk5/CIP* active conformations, then the protein pairs might not be able to interact anymore. One way to identify such cases is to measure the displacement of the template interface amino acids for a given conformation: if the displacement values are significant then the amino acids may not actually represent a protein interface. At such conformations the proteins are expected to dissociate, based on the

23

conservation hypothesis (see Figure 22). Also the distance function $D^k(\mathbf{T}^k A^k, B^k)$ defined in Equation (13) will provide a measure of the geometric affinity with no actual biochemical meaning, as the given protein pair is not expected to interact. Therefore, this is a useful geometric criterion for discarding geometric affinity values when the interface conformations are such that no interaction can be expected.

For a formal definition of the above described geometric criterion, recall that the distance function $D^k(\mathbf{T}^k A^k, B^k)$ defined in Equation (13) consists of the summation of second powers of the distances between 22 interface amino acid pairs and their corresponding ideal locations based on conservation hypothesis. Also the interface amino acids are identified as the ones having distance less than 3.5 Å from the other protein. Therefore, a threshold for the maximum allowed mean displacement of interface amino acids from their ideal position can be used as a displacement criterion (refer to Figure 22). It can be shown by simple mathematical formulae that the distance function value obtained from Equation (13) has the following relationship with the displacement threshold.

$$D^k < np * \zeta^2 \tag{21}$$

where D^k is the distance value obtained from the distance function $D^k(\mathbf{T}^k A^k, B^k)$ defined in Equation (13) for the k-th protein conformation pair, np is the number of interface amino acid pairs (22 in our case), and ζ is the chosen threshold value in terms of the mean displacement of interface amino acids from their ideal location. Inequality (21) represents the distance value above which the mean displacement of interface amino acids from their ideal position is so large that no significant protein interaction should occur, based on the conservation hypothesis. In this case the geometric affinity value has no meaning and can be discarded. For instance, setting a threshold of $\zeta = 1$ Å, from Equation (21) we would have a corresponding distance value of 22. Similarly, a threshold of $\zeta = 1.5$ corresponds to a distance value of 88. Considering that we used the 3.5 Å threshold to identify protein surfaces, a threshold of $\zeta \approx 1.8$ Å which corresponds to a distance value of ≈ 71 seems reasonable.

5.2 Results

The results of the comparison between the geometric affinities to *cdk5* of *p25* and *CIP* are presented in this section (refer to figures 23 to 29). Figure 23 shows the distance values from Equation (13), resulting from the application of the COMPUTEKTHDISTANCEFUNCTION algorithm to the *cdk5/p25* and *cdk5/CIP* conformations. The following *p25* and *CIP* conformations were investigated: $p25_i$ and CIP_i with $i = 0, 500, 1000, 1500, 2000, 2500, 3000$. Note that the distance values from Equation (13) for both *p25* and *CIP* go beyond the threshold value of ≈ 71 defined above. This means that the mean displacement of interface amino acids from their ideal location is greater than $\zeta \approx 1.8$. Based on the conservation hypothesis, the interface conformational changes are such that significant interactions should not be expected between *cdk5* and *p25* or *CIP* beyond. So in these cases the geometric affinity values for protein interfaces can be discarded. This is not surprising as both *p25* and *CIP* are expected to be significantly less flexible than *cdk5* and hence not to be able to follow *cdk5* conformational changes very far from

24

their active conformations. Figure 24 plots the distance values from Equation (13) vs. *p25* and *CIP* corresponding conformations on an expanded scale. The following *p25* and *CIP* conformations have been investigated: $p25_i$ and CIP_i with $i = 0, 50, 100, 150, 200, 250, 300, 350, 400, 450, 500$. Even in this case the distance values from Equation (13) for both *p25* and *CIP* go beyond the threshold value above defined of ≈ 71. Only $p25_i$ and CIP_i with $i < 50$ identify *p25* and *CIP* conformations that are expected to interact substantially with *cdk5*. For those conformations our technique will be able compare *p25* and *CIP* geometric affinity to *cdk5*.

Figure 25 is a plot of distance values from Equation (13) computed for several *p25* and *CIP* conformations. In this case the following *p25* and *CIP* conformations have been investigated: $p25_i$ and CIP_i with $i = 0, 10, 20, 30, 40, 50$. The distance values from Equation (13) for both *p25* and *CIP* are higher than the threshold value in correspondence of the 40th conformations $p25_{40}$ and CIP_{40}. Therefore we will focus on conformations between the active one and the 40th. As it can be noticed from Figure 25, there is a full *p25* and *CIP* conformation range between 20th conformation and 40th one such that *p25* distance values from Equation (13) are higher than *CIP* ones. This means that *CIP* geometric affinity is higher than *p25* for those conformations. Furthermore 10th to 20th conformation range values need to be checked. In fact in correspondence of 10th conformation *p25* distance value from Equation (13) is lower than *CIP*, but the opposite occurs in correspondence of 20th conformation. Hence, more detailed results about the range between active and 40th conformation are needed.

In Figure 26 the distance values from Equation (13) vs. *p25* and *CIP* corresponding conformations are shown for conformations $p25_i$ and CIP_i with $i = 10$ to 20. In the whole range except for the 10th conformation *CIP* distance values are clearly lower than for *p25*. This means that *CIP* geometric affinity is higher than *p25* one for those conformations. Same holds for Figure 27, where distance values from Equation (13) vs. *p25* and *CIP* corresponding conformations are shown for conformations $p25_i$ and CIP_i with $i = 20$ to 30. In this case *CIP* distance values are lower than for *p25* for the whole range. Finally, in Figure 28 distance values from Equation (13) vs. *p25* and *CIP* corresponding conformations are shown for conformations $p25_i$ and CIP_i with $i = 30$ to 40. As observed above, conformations 36th to 40th for both *CIP* and *p25* have distance values higher than the threshold. For the remaining distance values we still see that *CIP* distance values are lower than for *p25*: *CIP* geometric affinity is higher than *p25* for those conformations.

From figures 26 to 28 we observe that, in compliance with the flexibility hypothesis, *CIP* conformations seem to be more geometrically affine to *cdk5* conformations then *p25* ones. Geometric affinity has been evaluated by using the distance function defined in Equation (13), which is based on the difference between *p25*/*CIP* interface amino acid current location and their ideal location. The ideal location is the location interface amino acids would have if they were interacting exactly as they were doing in the crystallized *cdk5*/*p25* active complex, in compliance with the conservation hypothesis. The ideal location has been defined based on the closest amino acid atoms, as well as the unique geometric representation of the relative position and orientation of the interface amino acid pairs, defined by the vector $K_i^0 = \left(\alpha_i^0, \beta_i^0, \gamma_i^0, d_{xi}^0, d_{yi}^0, d_{zi}^0 \right) \forall i = 1, ..., 22$ from Equation (4). Hence, the geometric affinity evaluation problem is efficiently addressed as a feature alignment problem with a decreased number of degrees of freedom involved.

Additional insights on protein interface relative orientations are also given. In Figure 29(a) to (c) plots referring to interface amino acid relative angle values α, β and γ from Equation (4) for a few *p25* or *CIP* conformations are shown. These angle values represent *p25* or

25

CIP interface amino acid orientation with respect to *cdk5*, as defined in Section 4.2.1. Let us define α_i^j, β_i^j and $\gamma_i^j \ \forall i = 1,...,22$ as the angles for the *j*-th *p25* or *CIP* conformation and α_i^o, β_i^o and $\gamma_i^o \ \forall i = 1,...,22$ as the angles for the active *p25* or *CIP* conformation. Then, the plots in Figure 29(a) to (c) show, respectively, for a given conformation *j* the following values:

$$\Delta \alpha_j = \sum_{i=1}^{22} \left| \alpha_i^j - \alpha_i^o \right|, \Delta \beta_j = \sum_{i=1}^{22} \left| \beta_i^j - \beta_i^o \right| \text{ and } \Delta \gamma_j = \sum_{i=1}^{22} \left| \gamma_i^j - \gamma_i^o \right| . \qquad \text{The angle values}$$

α_i^j, β_i^j and $\gamma_i^j \ \forall i = 1,...,22$ are computed after performing the alignment through algorithm COMPUTEKTHDISTANCEFUNCTION. In particular *p25* and *CIP* conformations $p25_i$ and CIP_i with *i* = 0, 10, 20, 30, 40, 50 have been considered. Note that for both α and γ the trend is similar to the distance values from Equation (13): *CIP* angle values are closer to the active conformations than *p25* ones. As for β case, *p25* angle values are slightly closer to the active conformations than *CIP* ones, but there is no significant difference as these values are obtained as a summation over all the 22 amino acid pairs. Therefore, these plots referring more directly to relative interface amino acid orientations seem not to go against the above results. Hence, we can infer that a few *CIP* conformations seem to be more geometrically affine to *cdk5* conformations than *p25* ones, in compliance with our flexibility hypothesis.

5.3 Discussion of results

Our results should be interpreted in light of the following issues.

- **Steric clashes between atoms.** Observe that in calculating the geometric affinity each amino acid residue is treated as a rigid body, and the corresponding alignment is obtained based on one set of coordinates per amino acid location. Thus there is no direct control on the orientation of non-interface residues or to side chains of interface residues. Therefore an alignment yielding an apparently high geometric affinity value between two interfaces may actually cause a number of steric clashes (see Figure 30). Hence, steric clashes between atoms should be analyzed before accepting the obtained geometric affinity values.

  However, the presence of some clashes after an alignment does not necessarily mean that the corresponding interface affinity value needs to be discarded. In fact the rigid side chain atoms might just need a little readjusting after the rigid alignment. Therefore, alignments with few clashes involving only a few side chain atoms can be still considered significant.

  For example, consider the 20th configuration of *cdk5*, *p25* and *CIP* in figures 31 and 32. As we can see, the protein alignment in the figure causes some atom clashes. If we focus on the atom clashes in detail, we realize that they involve side chain amino acids that can easily readjust in order not to cause clashes anymore, without significantly affecting the geometric affinity measure. In fact, even if the amino acid side chains that are readjusted involved atoms representing the protein interface, their displacement resulting from side chain adjustment would be usually so small that the overall geometric affinity value would not change significantly. In figures 31 and 32 the protein alignment after eliminating the clashes is shown, with particular focus on the affected side chains. The readjustment has been obtained by using the molecular dynamics software NAMD [Kal99]. Protein atoms were kept fixed in space except for the clashing side chains, which were left free to move and readjust. This way a minimum energy configuration was reached without significantly affecting the obtained alignment. The corresponding distance values are shown: there are no significant changes as anticipated. Therefore *CIP* has still higher geometric affinity than *p25* based on the distance values.

Hence, as long as the small number of clashes can be eliminated as in the above-described case, the corresponding geometric affinity value is still significant. We have checked a few of the obtained protein alignments by the above procedure based on the software NAMD. We focused on the range between the 10th protein conformations and the 36th protein conformations, where *CIP* geometric affinity to *cdk5* seems to always be higher than *p25*. For all of them very few or no clashes were identified and they were easily eliminated without significantly affecting the geometric affinity values. This could be expected just looking at the protein alignments (Figure 33): all of them involve protein conformations that are very close to the active complex *cdk5/p25*. Therefore no major clashes are expected upon alignment. On the other hand protein conformations that are very different from the active complex *cdk5/p25* cannot be handled similarly. In fact in the figure an instance of alignment of conformation 2000 is also shown: in this case the protein conformations are very different from the active *cdk5/p25* complex and therefore there are many clashes that cannot be fixed by just allowing simple readjustments of the side chains. So in conclusion the geometric affinity values for the protein conformations of our interest are significant and can be used to verify the flexibility hypothesis.

- **Assessment of active/inactive state for given *cdk5* conformations.** A range of *cdk5*, *p25* and *CIP* conformations has been identified that seems to show that *CIP* has higher geometric affinity to *cdk5* than *p25* has to *cdk5*. This suggests that *CIP* might bind to *cdk5* more easily than *p25* does in correspondence of these conformations. However, in order for *CIP* to bind to *cdk5* and therefore prevent *p25* from activating *cdk5* (i.e. flexibility hypothesis), the binding has to involve inactive *cdk5* conformations (see Figure 34). This means that there must be at least a few *cdk5* conformations from the identified range that are still inactive. Observe that *cdk5* is not expected to suddenly become inactive, but a few conformations, very close to the crystallized one, are expected to be still active. Then, as *cdk5* main elements significantly change location/orientation, *cdk5* will become inactive at some point. Therefore it would be important to identify the *cdk5* conformations that are expected to be active among the ones from the above-mentioned range.

  For other cyclin-dependent kinases such as *cdk2*/cyclin complex the activation mechanism has already been studied in detail [Bro95]. Therefore, similarly to when we obtained *cdk5* inactive conformation, we use *cdk2* as model. From [Bro95] it can be inferred that very small conformational changes are expected to inactivate *cdk2*. In particular, a few *cdk2* and cyclin amino acids are identified, whose relative locations cannot change significantly in order for *cdk2* to stay active. Hence, in order to evaluate if a given *cdk5* conformation is expected to be active, we refer to the corresponding significant amino acid positions in *cdk5/p25* complex. By homology with *cdk2*/cyclin complex, the hyperphosphorylation of other proteins can only occur if *cdk5/p25* complex binds to the protein to be hyperphosphorylated (i.e. substrate) as well as to ATP in a very specific way. A few significant *cdk5/p25* complex amino acids are identified as follows.

  Let us consider the active *cdk5/p25* complex shown in Figure 35(a). Based on [Bro95] and on our knowledge of *cdk5* function in the brain, there are two regions of interest in *cdk5/p25* complex. They are the binding pocket for ATP and the binding site for the substrate protein to be phosphorylated. As it is shown in the figure, we chose three amino acids to represent the above-mentioned regions. Amino acids GLU 240 from *p25* (in purple) and ASP 126 from *cdk5* (in red) represent *cdk5* and *p25* regions that bind to the substrate. In fact ASP 126 is supposed to bind to a particular amino acid of the substrate and keep it in the right location to be phosphorylated. On the other hand GLU 240 is an amino acid from *p25* that is likely to interact with the substrate, holding its last amino acid in place. Finally GLU 81 (in green) represents *cdk5* binding pocket for ATP. So these three selected amino acids, represented by Van Der Waals spheres in the figure, are significant for *cdk5* activation. In Figure 35(b) the relative distances are shown for the active complex. As observed above, in order for a given protein conformation to be active the three amino acid relative locations need to be conserved very precisely with respect to the fully active protein complex. To verify this, we have focused on a few representative *cdk5* and *p25* conformations, so as to check if there were significant changes in the relative locations of these three amino acids. The proteins were first aligned by using the above-described COMPUTEKTHDISTANCEFUNCTION algorithm. In Figure 36 only the three amino acids of interest are shown upon each alignment for the following *cdk5* and *p25* conformations: $cdk5_i$ and $p25_i$ with $i = 10, 20, 30, 40$. As we can see from the figure, for the 10th conformation the relative distances are still very close to the active conformation ones, suggesting that the complex is likely to be active. As can be observed in Figure 36 (b)-(c)-(d), all three distances generally increase. In particular, the one between ASP 126 of cdk5 and GLU 240 of *p25* significantly increases, suggesting that the substrate might be displaced in such a way that no phosphorylation would be possible anymore, as both the amino acids are supposed to interact with the substrate. In addition, the distance between GLU 81 and ASP 126 is also slightly increasing, suggesting that the relative position between ATP and the substrate might not be anymore suitable for phosphorylation. Therefore, if we consider the need of a very precise binding in order for *cdk5/p25* complex to be active, starting from the 20th *cdk5* and *p25* conformations we start seeing significant changes in the distance values. Therefore, based on these observations, it is reasonable to expect that somewhere in the range between 20th and 30th conformations *cdk5* inactivation may occur. However, we are aware that it will be necessary to use molecular dynamics simulations to study more accurately *cdk5* activation/inactivation process; we are currently pursuing this.

Finally, based also on the two items discussed above, the outcome of the comparison between *p25* and *CIP* geometric affinity to *cdk5* corresponding conformations can be interpreted as follows. We identified a range of *cdk5*, *p25* and *CIP* conformations that seems to show, based on conservation hypothesis, that *CIP* has higher geometric affinity to *cdk5* than *p25*. So *CIP* is expected to bind to *cdk5* more easily than *p25* for these conformations. We also observed, based on [Bro95] and on our knowledge of *cdk5* function, that a few *cdk5* conformations from the identified range might be inactive. Therefore *CIP* seems to be able to bind to *cdk5* inactive conformations and therefore prevent *p25* from binding and activating them. This complies with our flexibility hypothesis. In the next section we draw the conclusions about this work and illustrate future directions.

6 CONCLUSIONS AND FUTURE WORK

Experimental studies, which are described in [Ami02], provided evidence that small truncations of *p35* produce a high-affinity inhibitor protein called *CIP*. These results are of fundamental importance for neurodegenerative diseases such as Alzheimer's, which are known to be associated with hyperphosphorylation of specific neuronal proteins. In this paper the binding mechanism of *cdk5-p25* and *cdk5-CIP* complexes has been studied in order to gain a better insight on the inhibitory activity of the protein *CIP*. Our *in silico* study is based on the conservation hypothesis, which asserts that at least part of the interface interaction for the crystallized *cdk5-p25* complex will be conserved for the other *cdk5-p25* and *cdk5-CIP* complex conformations. Our aim was to verify the flexibility hypothesis, which asserts that increased flexibility is induced by *p25*'s truncation to *CIP* which allows it to conform to the *cdk5* interface more fully and prevents *cdk5* from achieving its fully active conformation.

We were able to compare the interactions between the proteins at the atomic level by using a geometry-based alignment algorithm. This algorithm attempts to fully align two given protein conformations based on the conservation hypothesis. The protein interfaces are represented as sets of points representing in turn their interacting amino acids. The algorithm aligns the proteins such that their interfaces are interacting geometrically as similarly as possible to the interface of the crystallized complex. Our alignment algorithm can be potentially generalized to the cases in which the protein surfaces to be aligned need to satisfy certain geometric conditions following from biochemical considerations.

Based on the conservation hypothesis our results seem to verify the flexibility hypothesis. Furthermore, we have also studied the protein conformations, derived by the FIRST/FRODA software, in order to gain additional insight on the activation state of the *cdk5-p25* and *cdk5-CIP* complexes. The flexibility and conservation hypotheses as well as our observations on the activation of the *cdk5-p25* and *cdk5-CIP* complexes can now be used as the basis for MD (molecular dynamics) simulations. In general, simulating *cdk5-p25* and *cdk5-CIP* interactions seems to be a computationally challenging task due to the complexity of their structures. However, based on our current results, we can efficiently setup our MD simulations by focusing on particular aspects rather than trying to fully reproduce *in silico* what took place *in vitro*. Some potentially interesting MD simulations that we intend to pursue are listed as follows.

- Simulate *cdk5-p25* and *cdk5-CIP* interaction for conformations that are very close to the crystallized *cdk5-p25* complex, focusing on the behavior of specific amino acids from the interface, from the ATP binding pocket and from the substrate binding pocket, in order to infer substantial differences in the behavior of the two complexes.

- Simulate *cdk5-p25-substrate-ATP* and *cdk5-CIP-substrate-ATP* interactions for conformations that are very close to the crystallized *cdk5-p25* complex focusing on the activation status of the complexes.

- Simulate *cdk5-p25-substrate-ATP* and *cdk5-CIP-substrate-ATP* interactions for conformations that are very close to the crystallized *cdk5-p25* complex after mutating some amino acids that we have identified as significant for the *cdk5* interaction with *p25* and *CIP* and for ATP and substrate binding.

These and additional MD simulations can now be more efficiently setup. In fact we identified several amino acids that seem to be more significant than others for *cdk5* interaction with *p25* and *CIP* and for *cdk5* activation. Also, our results indicates that the phenomena of interest occurs very close to the crystalized *cdk5-p25* conformation. Therefore we expect MD simulations to provide useful insights on *cdk5* conformations close to the crystallized forms, which will involve much less computational effort. Also, the analysis of MD data can be performed by focusing on only a few significant amino acids. Both these will lead to more efficient MD simulations.

DISCLAIMER

Certain commercial software systems are identified in this paper. Such identification does not imply recommendation or endorsement by the National Institute of Standards and Technology (NIST); nor does it imply that the products identified are necessarily the best available for the purpose. Further, any opinions, findings, conclusions or recommendations expressed in this material are those of the authors and do not necessarily reflect the views of NIST or any other supporting US government or corporate organizations.

7 REFERENCES

[Aba94a]   R. A. Abagyan, M. M. Totrov, and D. A. Kuznetsov. ICM: a new method for protein modeling and design: applications to docking and structure prediction from the distorted native conformation. *Journal of Computational Chemistry*, 15(5): 488-506, 1994.

[Aba94b]   R.A. Abagyan, and M. M. Totrov. Biased probability Monte Carlo conformational searches and electrostatic calculations for peptides and proteins. *Journal of Molecular Biology*, 235(3): 983-1002, 1994.

[Aga03a]   P. Agarwal, S. Krishnan, N. H. Mustafa, and S. Venkatasubramanian. Streaming geometric optimization using graphics hardware. In Proceedings of *11th Annual European Symposium On Algorithms*, 2003.

[Aga03b]   P. Agarwal, S. Har-Peled, M. Sharir, and Y. Wang. Hausdorff distance under translations of points, disks, and balls. In Proceeding Of 19th *Annual ACM Symposium On Computational Geometry*, 282-291, 2003.

[Alt88]   H. Alt, K. Mehlhorn, H. Wagener, and E. Welzl. Congruence, similarity and symmetries of geometric objects. *Discrete And Computational Geometry*, 3: 237-256, 1988.

[Alt96]   H. Alt and L.J. Guibas. Discrete geometric shapes: matching, interpolation, and approximation: a survey. *Technical Report B96-11, EVL-1996-142*, Institute of Computer Science, Freie Universität Berlin, December 1996.

[Ami02]   N. D. Amin, W. Albers, and H. C. Pant. Cyclin-dependent kinase 5 (cdk5) activation requires interaction with three domains of p35. *Journal of Neuroscience Research*, 67: 354–362, 2002.

[And01]   I. Andricioaei, J. E. Straub, and A. F. Voter. Smart darting Monte Carlo. *Journal of Chemical Physics*, 114(16): 6994-7000, 2001.

[Ati01]   A. R. Atilgan, S. R. Durell, R. L. Jernigan, M. C. Demirel, O. Keskin, and I. Bahar. Anisotropy of fluctuation dynamics of proteins with an elastic network model. *Biophysics Journal*, 80(): 505-15, 2001.

[Atk87]   M. D. Atkinson. An optimal algorithm for geometrical congruence. *Journal Of Algorithms*, 8(2): 159-172, 1987.

[Bah05]   I. Bahar, A. J. Rader. Coarse-grained normal mode analysis in structural biology. *Current Opinion in Structural Biology*, 15(5):586-592, October 2005.

[Bar94]   V. Barbu. Mathematical Methods in Optimization of Differential Systems (Mathematics and Its Applications). *Springer*, December 1994.

[Bet99]   M. J. Betts, and M. J. Sternberg. An analysis of conformational changes on protein–protein association: implications for predictive docking. *Protein Engineering*, 12(4): 271–283, 1999.

[Bro95]   N. R. Brown, M. E. Noble, J. A. Endicott, E. F. Garman, S. Wakatsuki, E. Mitchell, B. Rasmussen, T. Hunt, L. N. Johnson. The crystal structure of cyclin A. *Structure*, 3(11):1131-1134, November 1995.

[Bur03]   B. Bursulaya, M. M. Totrov, R. A. Abagyan, and C. Brooks. Comparative study of several algorithms for flexible ligand docking. *Journal of Computer Aided Molecular Design*, 17(11): 755-763, 2003.

[Car03]   A. Cardone, S. K. Gupta, and M. Karnik. A Survey Of Shape Similarity Assessment Algorithms For Product Design And Manufacturing Applications. *Journal Of Computing And Information Science In Engineering*, 3(2):109-118, June 2003.

[Car04]   A. Cardone, S. K. Gupta, and M. Karnik. Identifying Similar Parts For Assisting Cost Estimation Of Prismatic Machined Parts. In Proceedings of *ASME 2004 Design Engineering Technical Conferences and Computer and Information in Engineering Conference*, Salt Lake City, Utah, USA, September 2004.

[Car06]   A. Cardone, S. K. Gupta, A. Deshmukh, and M. Karnik. Machining Feature-Based Similarity Assessment Algorithms For Prismatic Machined Parts. *Computer Aided Design*, 38(9): 954-972, September 2006.

[Cam01]   R. J. Campbell and P. J. Flynn. A Survey On Free-Form Object Representation And Recognition Techniques. *Computer Vision And Image Understanding*, 81(2): 166-210, February 2001.

[Cas05]   D. A. Case, T. Cheatham, T. Darden, H. Gohlke, R. Luo, K. M. Merz, A. Onufriev, C. Simmerling, B. Wang, and R. Woods. The Amber biomolecular simulation programs. *Journal of Computational Chemistry*, 26: 1668-1688, 2005.

[Che99]   L. P. Chew, D. Dor, A. Efrat, and K. Kedem. Geometric pattern matching in d dimensional space. *Discrete And Computational Geometry*, 21: 257-274, 1999.

[Con99]   L. L. Conte, C. Chothia, and J. Janin. The atomic structure of protein–protein recognition sites. *Journal of Molecular Biology*, 285(5): 2177–2198, 1999.

[Fer02]   J. Fernandez-Recon, M. Totrov, and R. Abagyan. Soft protein-protein docking in internal coordinates. *Protein Science*, 11(2): 280-291, February 2002.

[Gab97]   H. A. Gabb, R. M. Jackson, and M. J. Sternberg. Modelling protein docking using shape complementarity, electrostatics and biochemical information. *Journal of Molecular Biology*, 272(1): 106–120, 1997.

[Gup99]   S.K. Gupta and D.A. Bourne. Sheet Metal Bending: Generating Shared Setups. *Journal Of Manufacturing Science And Engineering*, 121(4): 689-694, November 1999.

[Hef94]   P. J. Heffernan and S. Schirra. Approximate decision algorithms for point set congruence. *Computational Geometry: Theory And Applications*, 4(3): 137-156, 1994.

[Hue07]   R. Huey, G. M. Morris, A. J. Olson, and D. S. Goodsell. A semiempirical free energy force field with charge-based desolvation. *Journal of Computational Chemistry*, 28: 1145-1152, 2007.

[Hum96]   W. Humphrey, A. Dalke, and K. Schulten. VMD: Visual molecular dynamics. *Journal of Molecular Graphics*, 14(1): 33-38, 1996.

[Hus02]   M. Huse, and J. Kuriyan. Conformational plasticity of protein kinases. *Cell*, 109(3):275-282, May 2002.

[Hut90]   D. Huttenlocher and S. Ullman. Recognizing solid objects by alignment with an image. *International Journal Of Computer Vision*, 5(2): 195-212, 1990.

[Hut92]   D. P. Huttenlocher, K. Kedem, and J. M. Kleinberg. On dynamic Voronoi diagrams and the minimum Hausdorff distance for point sets under Euclidean motion in the plane. In Proceedings of 8th *Annual ACM Symposium On Computational Geometry*, 110-120, 1992.

[Hut93a]   D. P. Huttenlocher, K. Kedem, and M. Sharir. The upper envelope of Voronoi surfaces and its applications. *Discrete And Computational Geometry*, 9: 267-291, 1993.

[Hut93b]   D. P. Huttenlocher and W. J. Rucklidge. A multi-resolution technique for comparing images using the Hausdorff distance. In Proceedings of *IEEE Conference In Computer Vision And Pattern Recognition*, 705-706, New York, NY, 1993.

[Hut93c]   D. P. Huttenlocher, G. A. Klanderman, and W. J. Rucklidge. Comparing images using the Hausdorff distance. *IEEE Transactions On Pattern Analysis And Machine Intelligence*, 15: 850-863, 1993.

[Iran96]   S. Irani and P. Raghavan. Combinatorial and experimental results for randomized point matching algorithms. In Proceedings of *12th Annual ACM Symposium On Computational Geometry*, 68-77, 1996.

[Iye05]   N. Iyer, S. Jayanti, K. Lou, Y. Kalyanaraman and K. Ramani. Shape-based searching for product lifecycle applications. *Computer Aided Design*, 37(13): 1435-1446, 2005.

[Jay05]   N. Iyer, S. Jayanti, K. Lou, Y. Kalyanaraman and K. Ramani. Three dimensional shape searching: state-of-the-art review and future trends. *Computer-Aided Design*, 37: 509–530, 2005.

[Jef95]   P. D. Jeffrey, A. A. Russo, K. Polyak, E. Gibbs, J. Hurwitz, J. Massagué, and N. P. Pavletich. Mechanism of CDK activation. *Nature*, 376(6538): 313-320, July 1995.

[Kal99]   L. Kale, R. Skeel, M. Bhandarkar, R. Brunner, A. Gursoy, N. Krawetz, J. Phillips, A. Shinozaki, K. Varadarajan, and K. Schulten. NAMD2: Greater scalability for parallel molecular dynamics. *Journal of Computational Physics*, 151, 283-312, 1999.

[Kar05]   M.V. Karnik, S.K. Gupta, and E.B. Magrab. Geometric Algorithms for Containment Analysis of Rotational Parts. *Computer Aided Design*, 37(2): 213-230, February 2005.

[Kra99]   B. Kramer, M. Rarey, and T. Lengauer. Evaluation of the flexx incremental construction algorithm for protein-ligand docking. *Proteins: Structure, Function, and Genetic*, 37(2):228–241, 1999.

[Lui00]   A. Luise, M. Falconi, and A. Desideri. Molecular dynamics simulation of solvated azurin: Correlation between surface solvent accessibility and water residence times. *Proteins*, 39(1): 56-67, 2000.

[Mor96]   G. M. Morris, D. S. Goodsell, R. Huey, and A. J. Olson. Distributed automated docking of flexible ligands to proteins: parallel applications of AutoDock 2.4. *Journal of Computer-Aided Molecular Design*, 10: 293-304, 1996.

[Mor98]   G. M. Morris, D. S. Goodsell, R. S. Halliday, R. Huey, W. E. Hart, R. K. Belew, and A. J. Olson. Automated docking using a Lamarckian genetic algorithm and empirical binding free energy function. *Journal of Computational Chemistry*, 19(14): 1639-1662, 1998.

[Mou99]   D. M. Mount, N. S. Netanyahu, and J. Le Moigne. Efficient algorithms for robust point pattern matching. *Pattern Recognition*, 32: 17-38, 1999.

[Mou01]   N. Mousseau, P. Derreumaux, G. T. Barkema, and R. Malek. Sampling activated mechanisms in proteins with the activation–relaxation technique. *Journal of Molecular Graphics*, 19(1): 78-86, 2001.

[Nor99]   R. Norel, D. Petrey, H. J. Wolfson, and R. Nussinov. Examination of shape complementarity in docking of unbound proteins. *Proteins*, 36(3): 307–317, 1999.

[Pal00]   P. N. Palma, L. Krippahl, J. E. Wampler, and J. J Moura. BiGGER: a new (soft) docking algorithm for predicting protein interactions. *Proteins*, 39(4): 372–384, 2000.

[Pav99]   N. P. Pavletich. Mechanisms of cyclin-dependent kinase regulation: structures of Cdks, their cyclin activators, and Cip and INK4 inhibitors. *Journal of Molecular Biology*, 287(5):821-828, April 1999.

[Ram01]   M. Ramesh, D. Yip-Hoi, and D. Dutta. Feature-Based Shape Similarity Measurement For Retrieval Of Mechanical Parts. *Journal Of Computing And Information Science In Engineering*, 1(3): 245-256, September 2001.

[Spr94]   J. Sprinzak and M. Werman. Affine point matching. *Pattern Recognition Letters*, 15(4): 337-339, 1994.

[Sur94]   M. C. Surles, J. S. Richardson, D. C. Richardson, and F. P. Brooks, Jr.. Sculpting proteins interactively: continual energy minimization embedded in a graphical modeling system. *Protein Science*, 3: 198-210, 1994.

[Tam00]   F. Tama F, F. X. Gadea, O. Marques, and Y. H. Sanejouand. Building-block approach for determining low-frequency normal modes of macromolecules. *Proteins*, 41(1): 1-7, 2000.

[Tam01]   F. Tama and Y. H. Sanejouand. Conformational change of proteins arising from normal mode calculations. *Protein Engineering*, 14(1): 1-6, 2001.

[Vaj04]   S. Vajda, and C. J. Camacho. Protein–protein docking: is the glass half-full or half-empty? *Trends in Biotechnology*, 22(3): 110-116, March 2004.

[Vel01]   R.C. Veltkmap. Shape matching: similarity measures and algorithms. In Proceedings of *International Conference On Shape Modeling And Applications*, Genova, Italy, May 2001.

[Ver03]   M. L. Verdonk, J. C. Cole, M. J. Hartshorn, C. W. Murray, and R. D. Taylor. Improved protein-ligand docking using GOLD. *Proteins*, 52(4): 609-623, 2003.

[Wel05]   S. Wells, S. Menor, B. Hespenheide, and M. F. Thorpe. Constrained geometric simulation of diffusive motion in proteins. *Physical Biology*, 2: S127-S136, 2005.

[Wolf97]   H.J. Wolfson and I. Rigoutsos. Geometric hashing: an overview. *IEEE Computational Science And Engineering*, 4:10-21, 1997.

[Yue90]   S. Y. Yue. Distance-constrained molecular docking by simulated annealing. *Protein Engineering*, 4(2): 177–184, 1990.

[Zhe05]   Y. L. Zheng, S. Kesavapany, M. Gravell, R. S. Hamilton, M. Schubert, N. Amin, W. Albers, P. Grant, and H. C. Pant. A Cdk5 inhibitory peptide reduces tau hyperphosphorylation and apoptosis in neurons. *The EMBO Journal*, 24: 209–220, 2005.

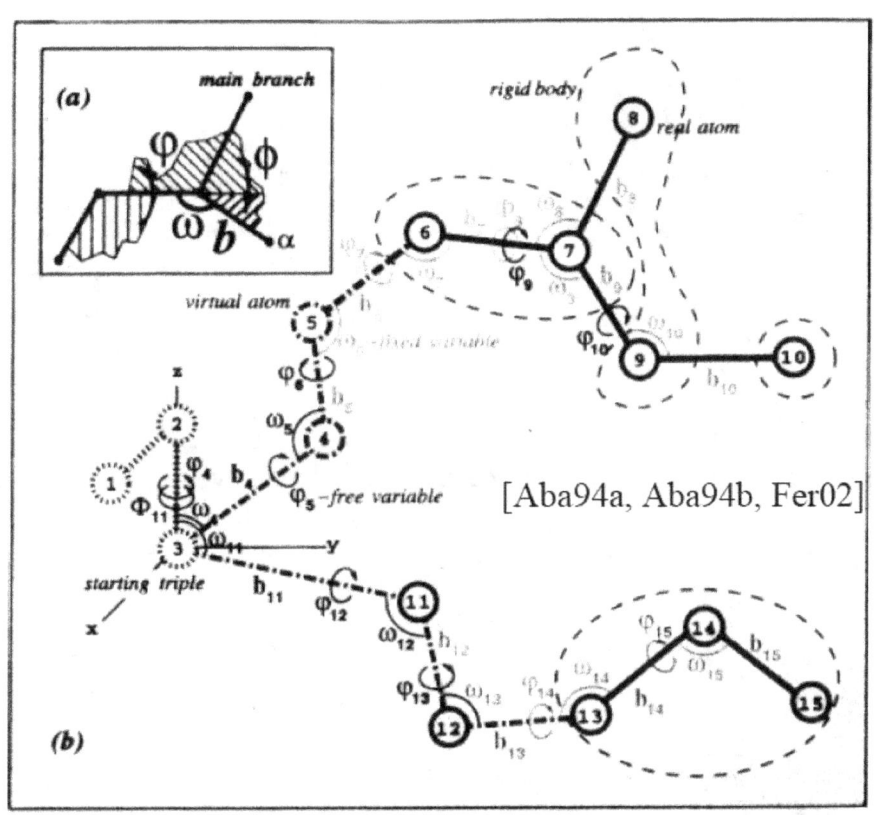

Figure 1. ICM technique is based on Internal Coordinate Mechanics

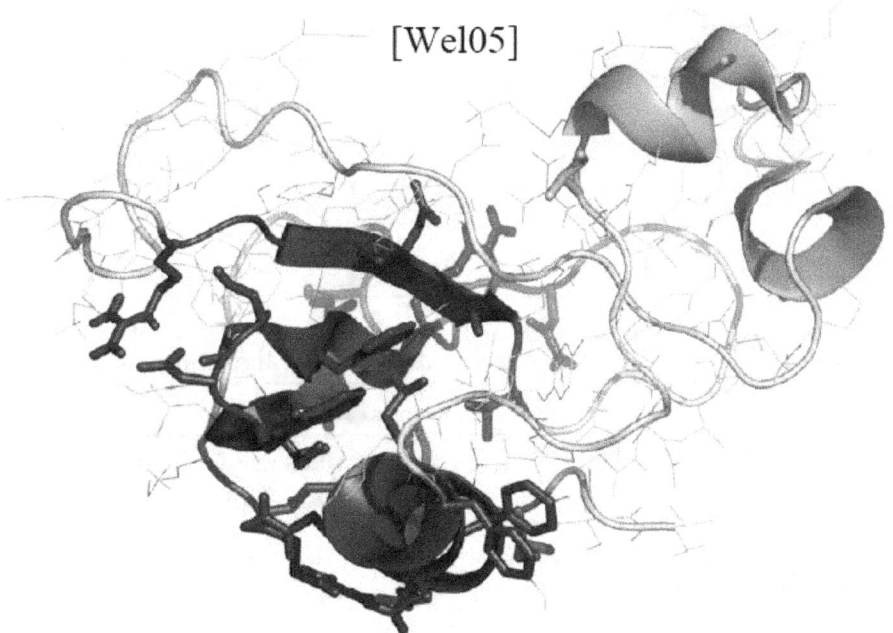

Figure 2. An example of rigid cluster decomposition by FIRST

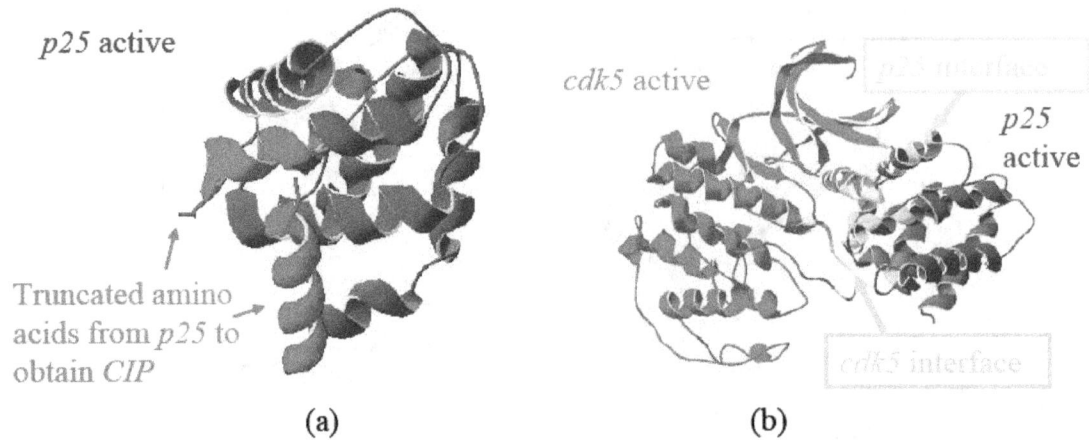

p25 active

Truncated amino
acids from *p25* to
obtain *CIP*

cdk5 active

p25
active

p25 interface

cdk5 interface

(a)   (b)

Figure 3.(a) *p25* truncation; (b) interface residues from active *cdk5/p25* complex

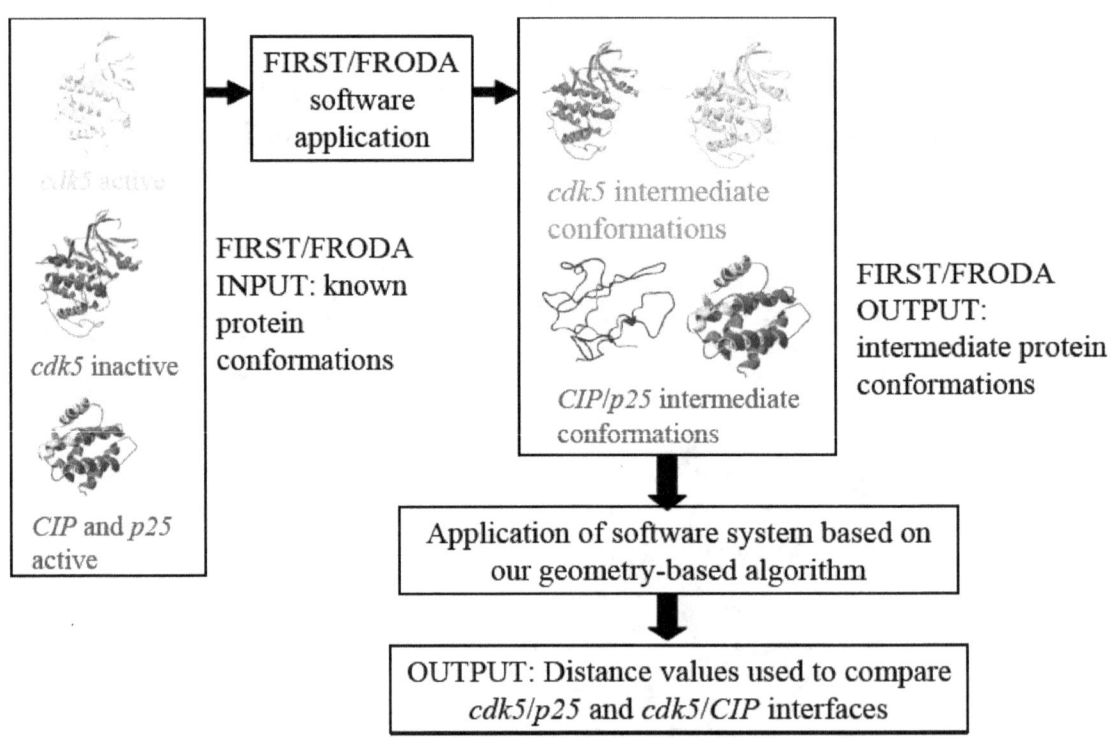

FIRST/FRODA
software
application

cdk5 active

cdk5 inactive

CIP and *p25*
active

FIRST/FRODA
INPUT: known
protein
conformations

cdk5 intermediate
conformations

CIP/p25 intermediate
conformations

FIRST/FRODA
OUTPUT:
intermediate protein
conformations

Application of software system based on
our geometry-based algorithm

OUTPUT: Distance values used to compare
cdk5/p25 and *cdk5/CIP* interfaces

Figure 4. Overview of our geometry-based technique to study *cdk5/p25* and *cdk5/CIP*
intermediate conformations

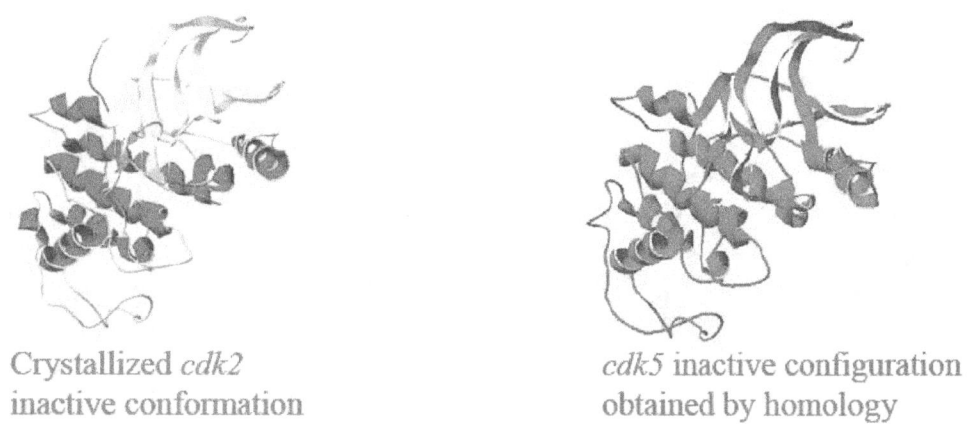

Crystallized *cdk2*
inactive conformation

cdk5 inactive configuration
obtained by homology

Figure 5. *Cdk5* inactive conformation is obtained by homology to the very similar crystalized *cdk2* inactive conformation

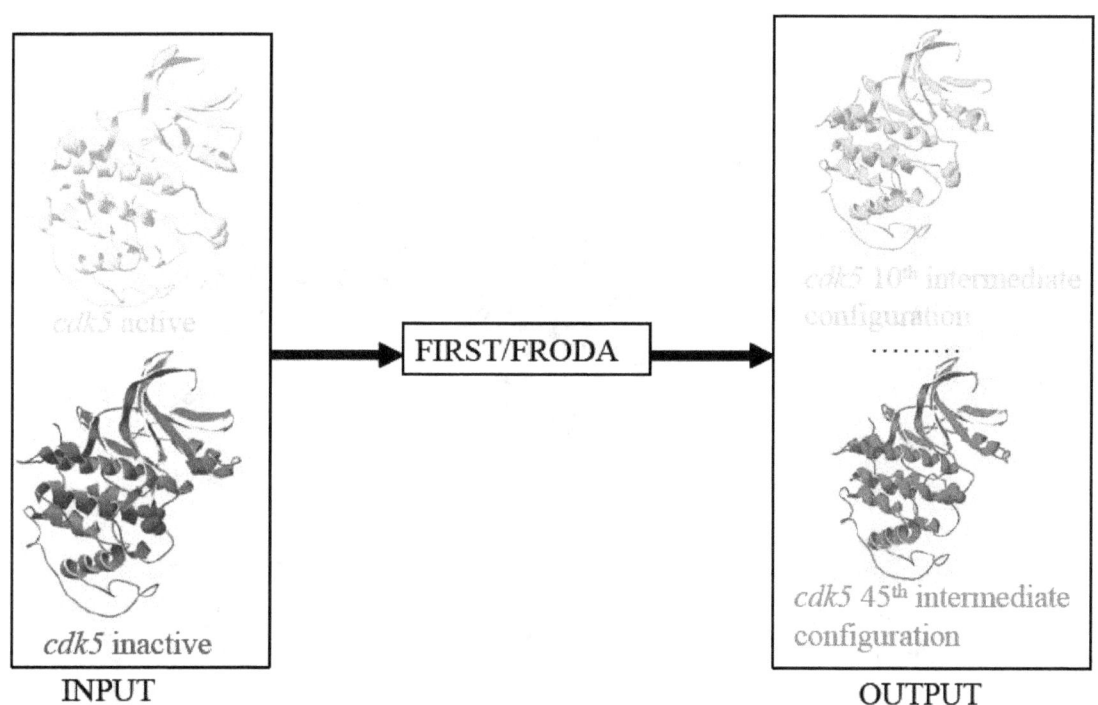

INPUT

OUTPUT

Figure 6. Instances of *cdk5* conformations obtained from FIRST/FRODA software

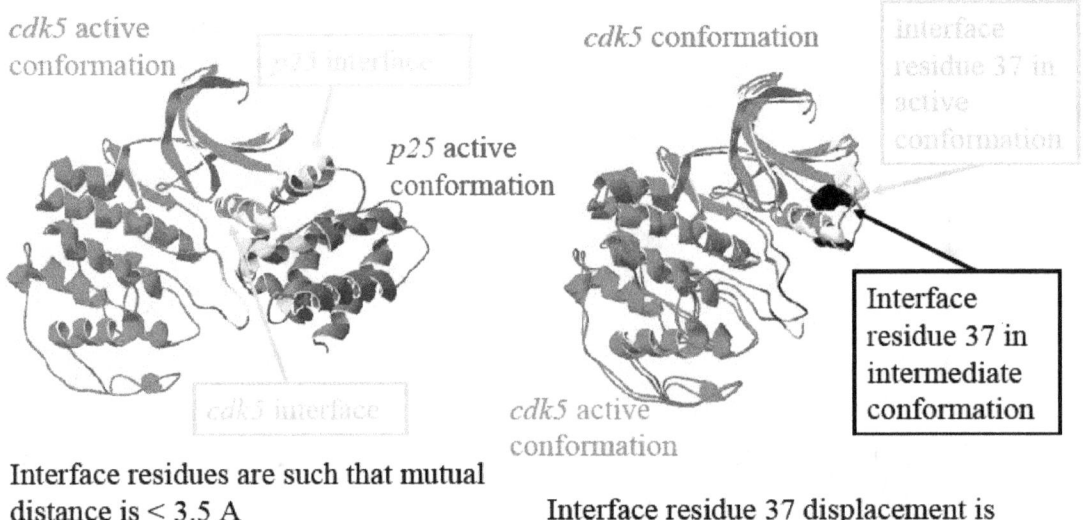

Interface residues are such that mutual distance is < 3.5 A

Interface residue 37 displacement is identified

Figure 7. Active *cdk5/p25* complex with interface residues and residue 37 displacement corresponding to a given *cdk5* conformation

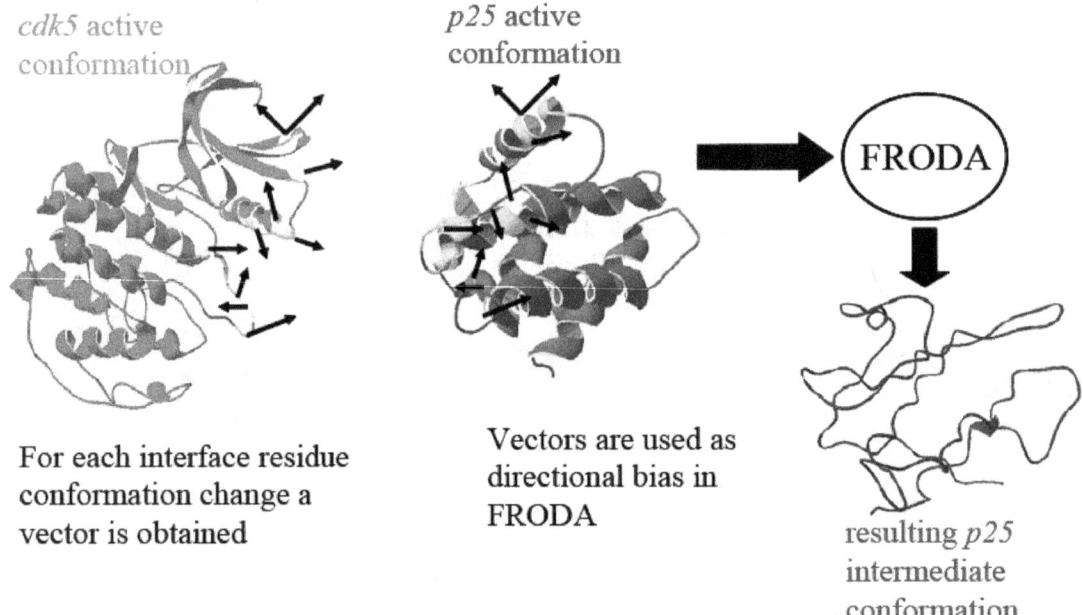

For each interface residue conformation change a vector is obtained

Vectors are used as directional bias in FRODA

resulting *p25* intermediate conformation

Figure 8. Vector representation of the *cdk5* interface conformational changes and corresponding *p25* conformation obtained by using FIRST/FRODA

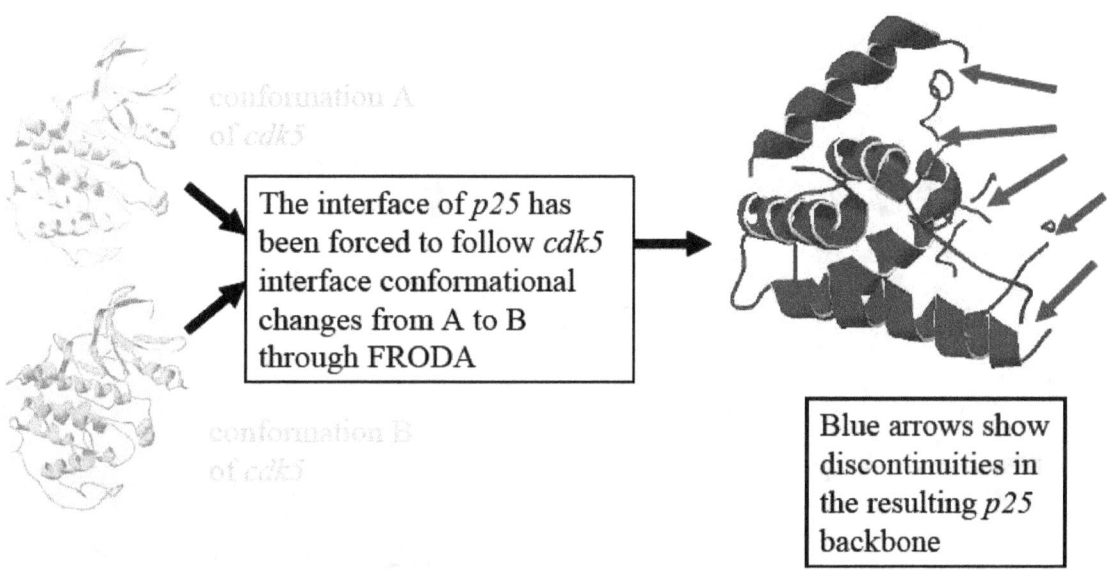

Figure 9. *P25* conformation resulting from the application of FRODA shows discontinuities in the backbone

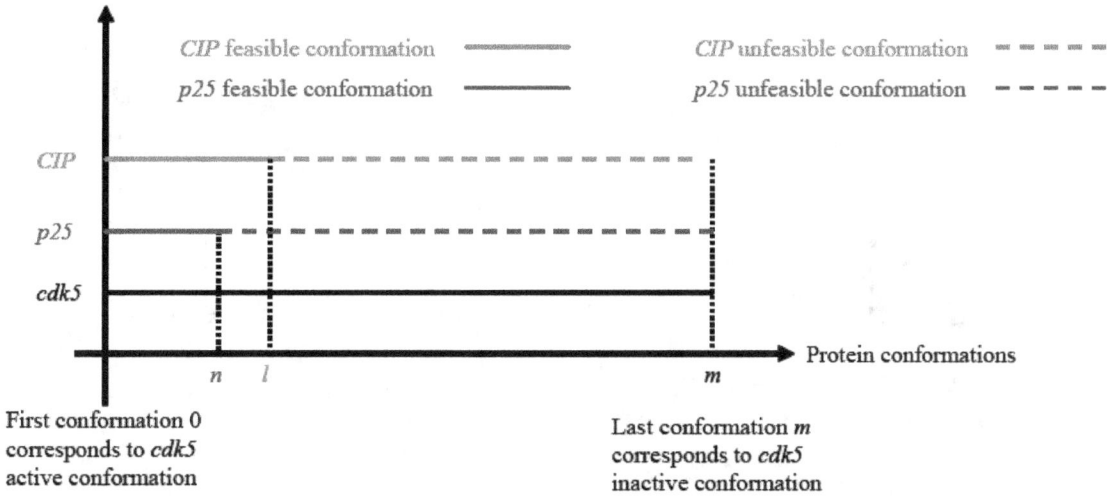

Figure 10. Plot representing *cdk5*, *p25* and *CIP* conformation obtained through FRODA

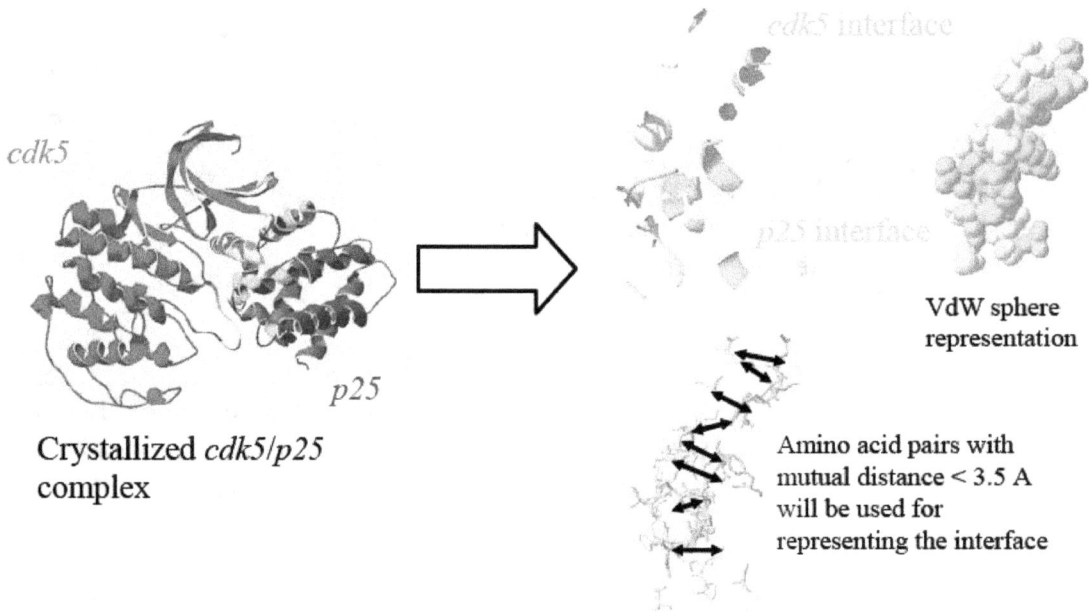

VdW sphere
representation

Crystallized *cdk5/p25*
complex

Amino acid pairs with
mutual distance < 3.5 A
will be used for
representing the interface

Figure 11. *cdk5/p25* complex interface and its representation

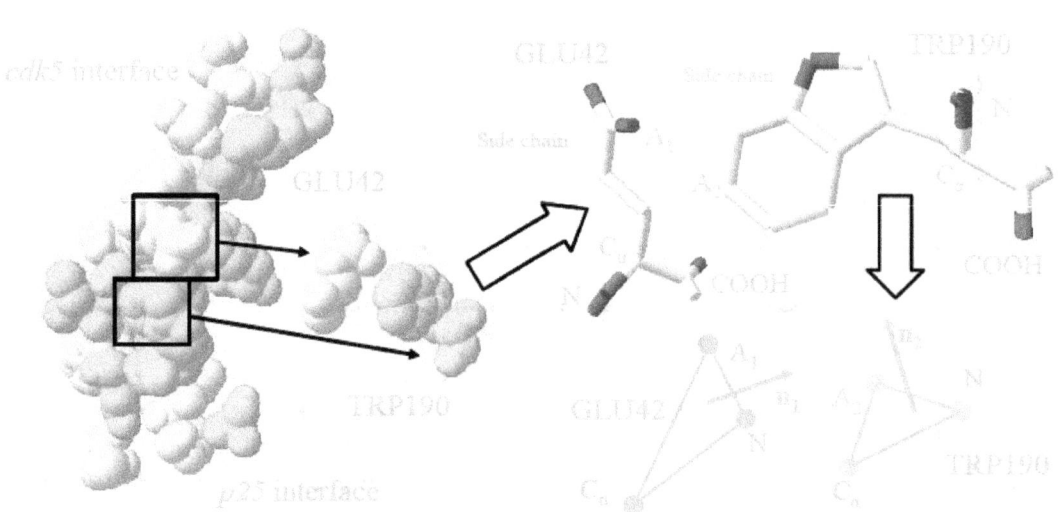

Figure 12. interacting amino acids GLU42 and TRP190 from *cdk5/p25* crystal interface

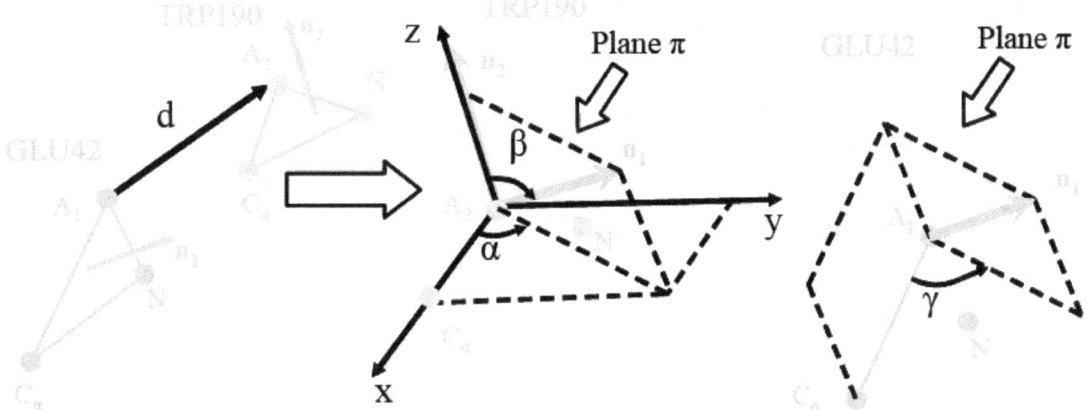

Relative position/orientation between GLU42 and TRP190 is function of α, β, γ and $d=(d_x, d_y, d_z)$

Figure 13. The six independent parameters that univocally represent the relative position and orientation of amino acid pair GLU42/TRP190 from *cdk5/p25* crystallized complex

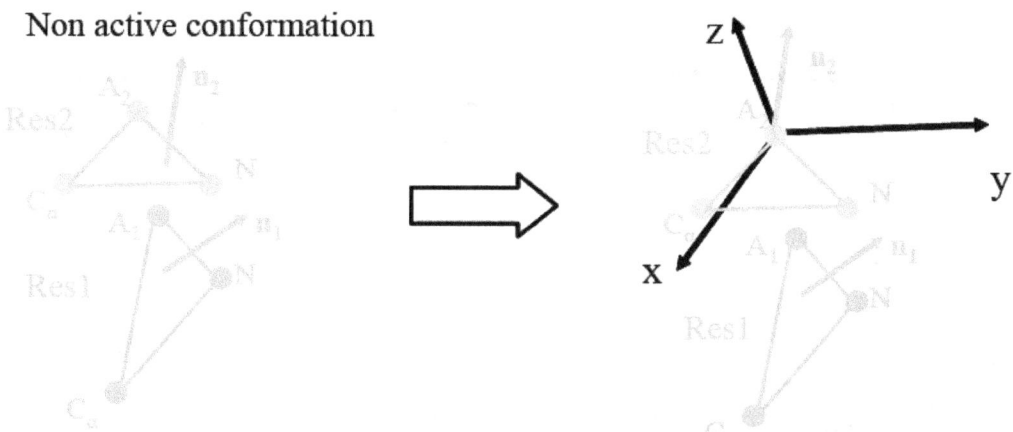

(a) Translation of both amino acids such that A_2 lies on the origin

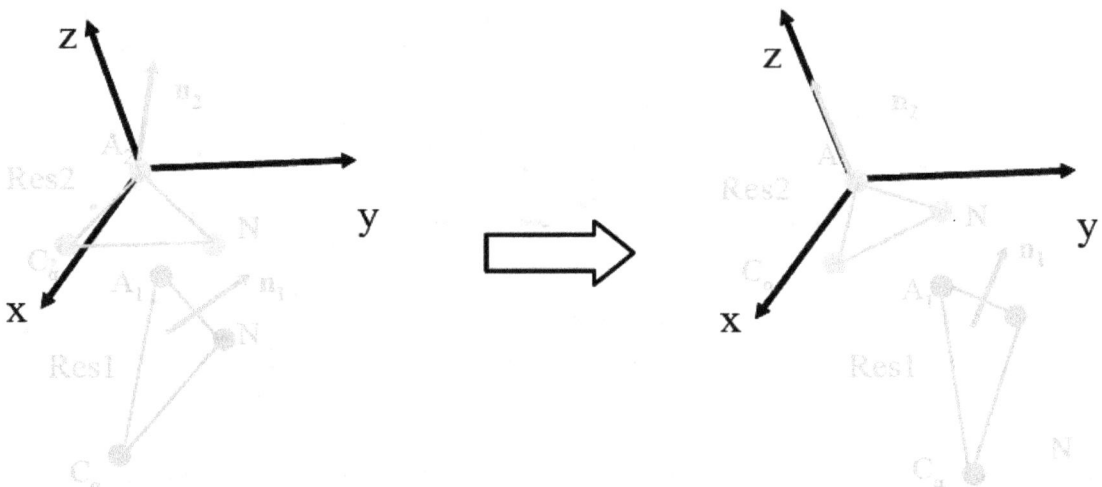

(b) Rotation of both amino acids such that n_2 is aligned to Z-axis

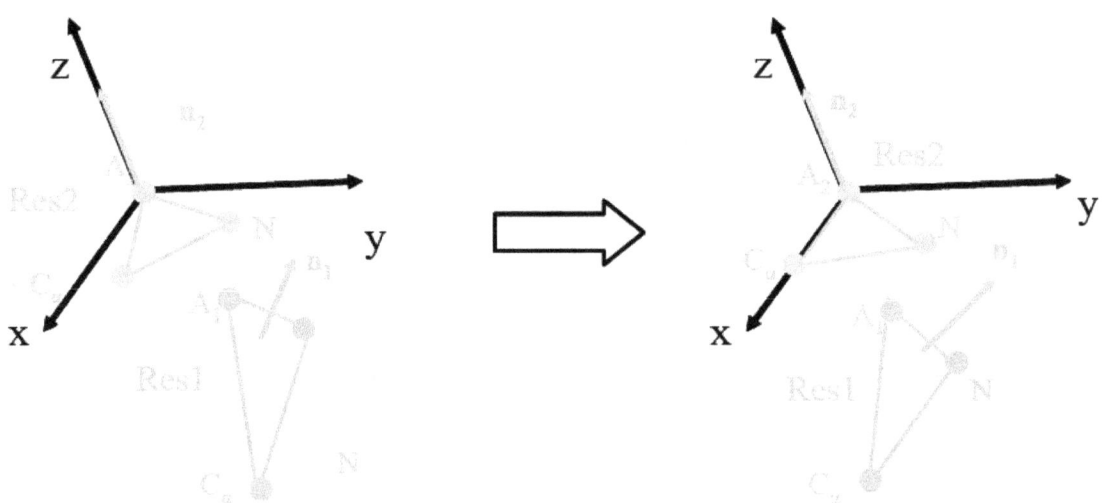

(c) Rotation of both amino acids such that C_α lies on X-axis

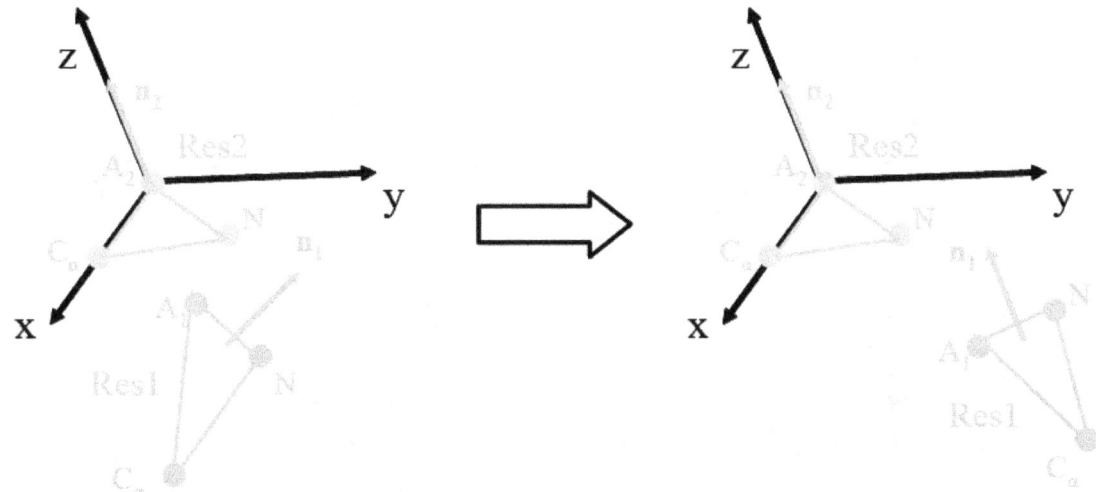

(d) Rotation of amino acid Res1 such that n_1 is aligned to Z-axis

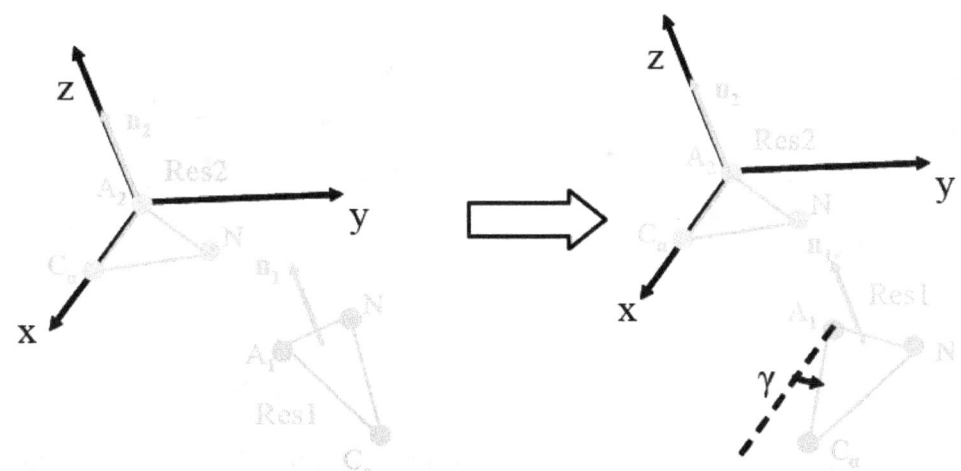

(e) Rotation of amino acid Res1 such that $C_\alpha A_1$ has an angle equal to γ with X-axis

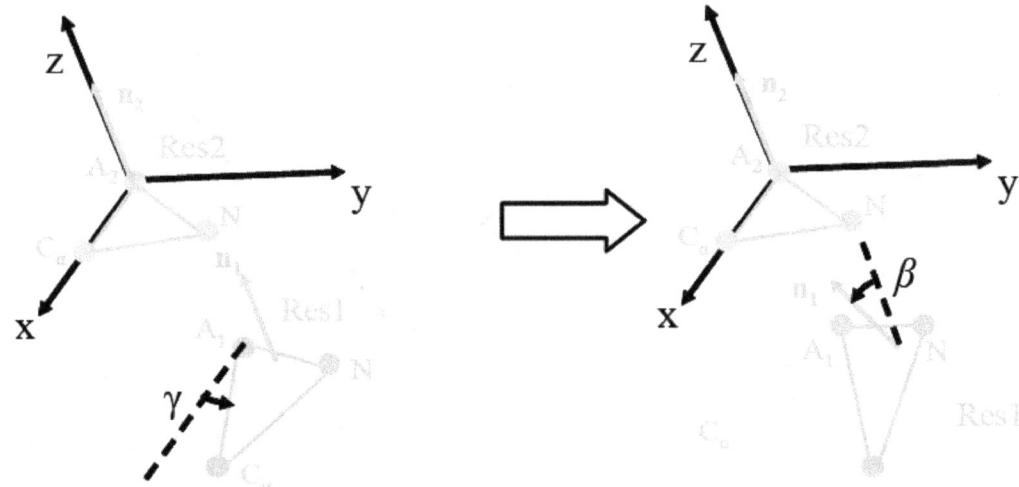

(f) Rotation of amino acid Res1 such that n_1 has an angle equal to β with Z-axis

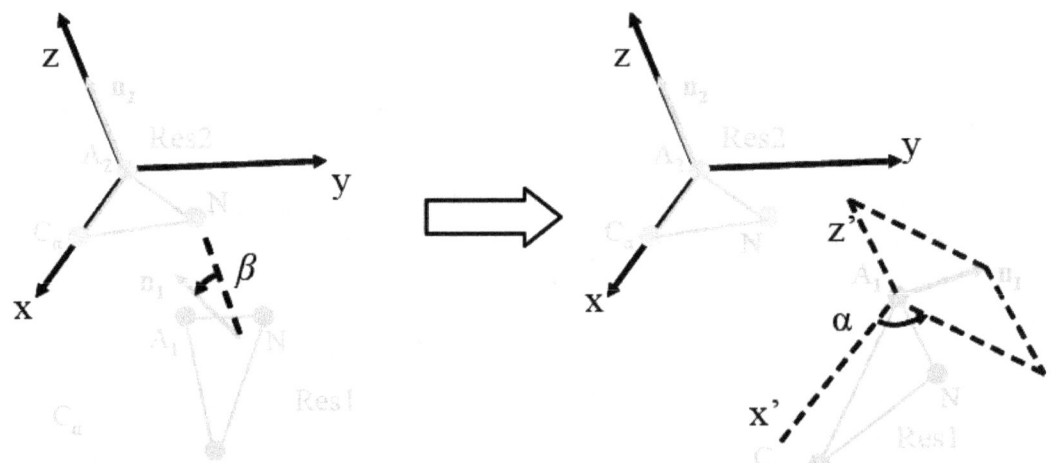

(g) Rotation of amino acid Res1 such that n_1 projection onto XY-plane has an angle equal to α with X-axis

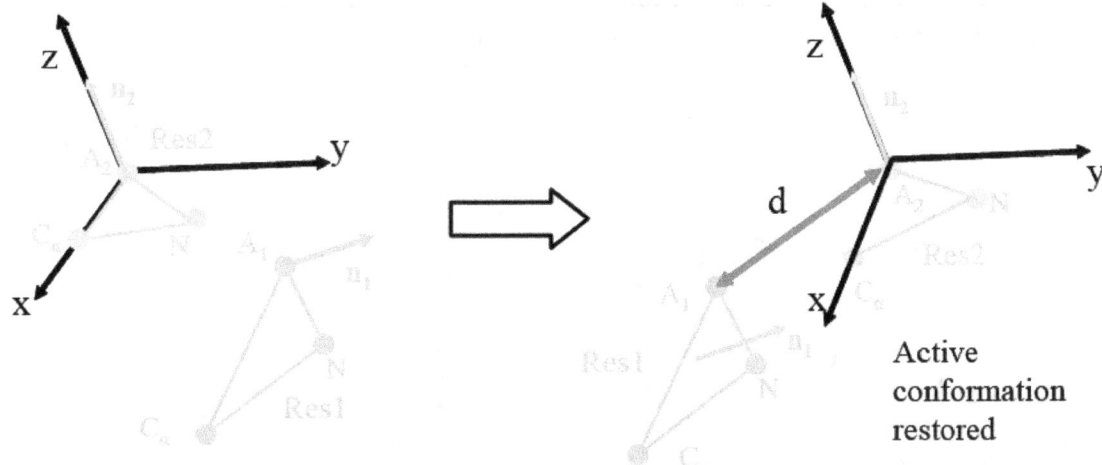

(h) Translation of amino acid Res1 such that A_1 is at distance d from the origin

Figure 14. Example of transformations described in steps 1 to 8 from ALIGN_RES_PAIR algorithm

2 DOF transformation space for point p_i: any point (x,y) represents a transformation T=(x,y) applied to point p_i

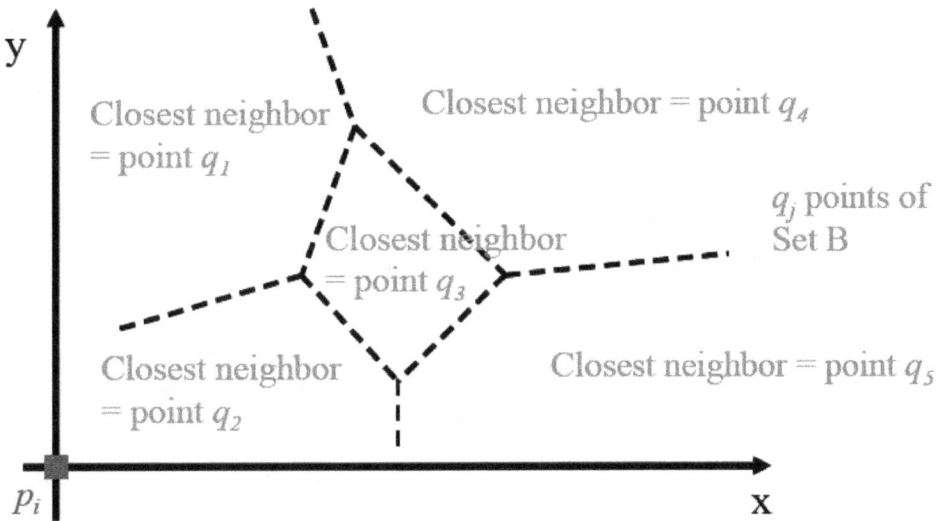

Figure 15. For each transformation T=(x,y) belonging to the same cell the resulting closest neighbor to point p_i from set B does not change

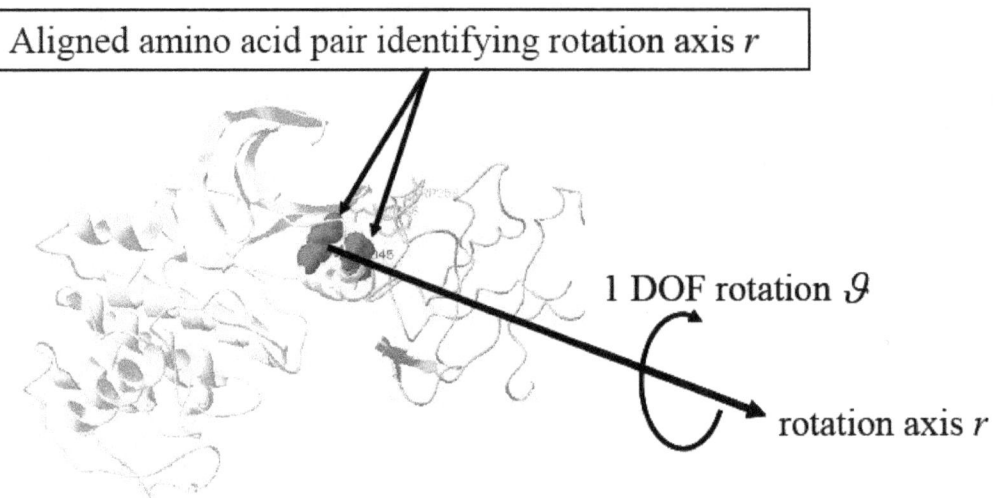

Figure 16. One degree of freedom rotation of protein *p25* around *r* axis which is identified by the aligned amino acid pair shown

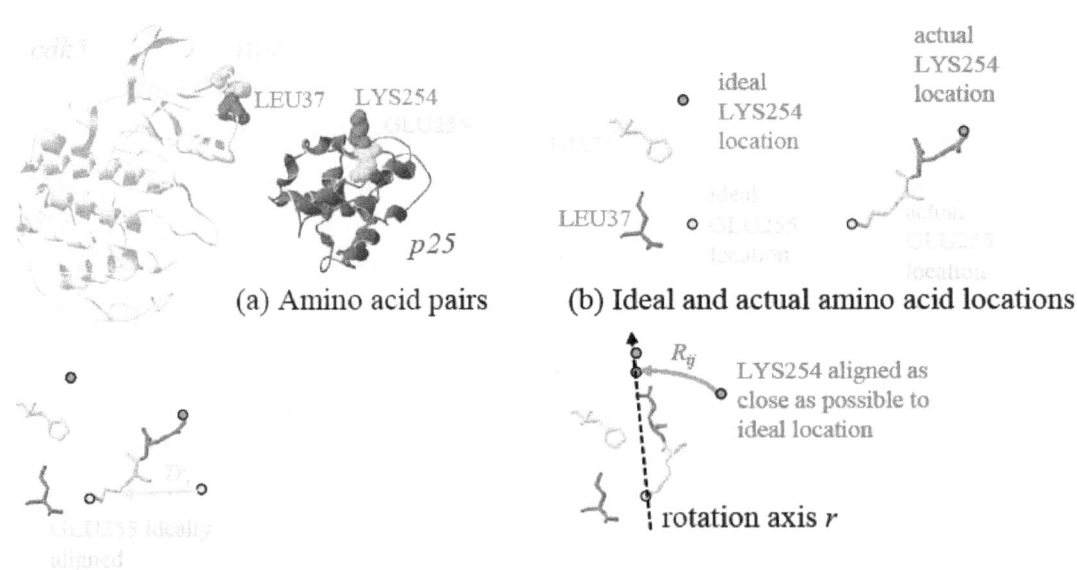

(a) Amino acid pairs   (b) Ideal and actual amino acid locations

(c) Translation Tr_i to ideally align GLU255   (d) Rotation R_{ij} to ideally align LYS254

Figure 17. Instance of amino acid pair alignment in the case of non coincident ideal locations

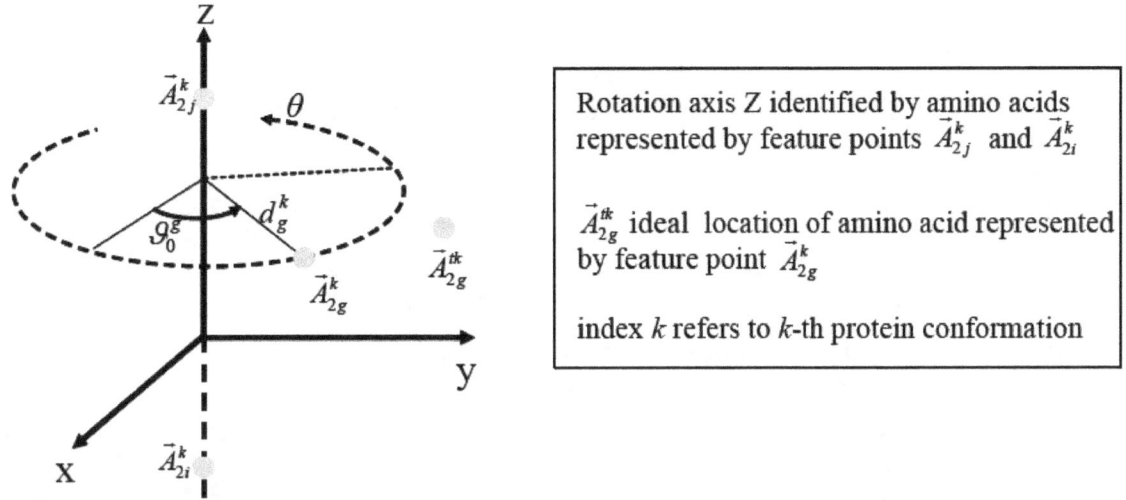

$\begin{cases} d_g^k = \text{constant distance of point } \vec{A}_{2g}^k \text{ from rotation axis corresponding to Z - axis} \\ \vartheta_0^g = \text{initial angle between the projection of } \vec{A}_{2g}^k \text{ onto coordinate plane XY and X - axis} \end{cases}$

Figure 19. Instance of geometric parameters used in distance function evaluation

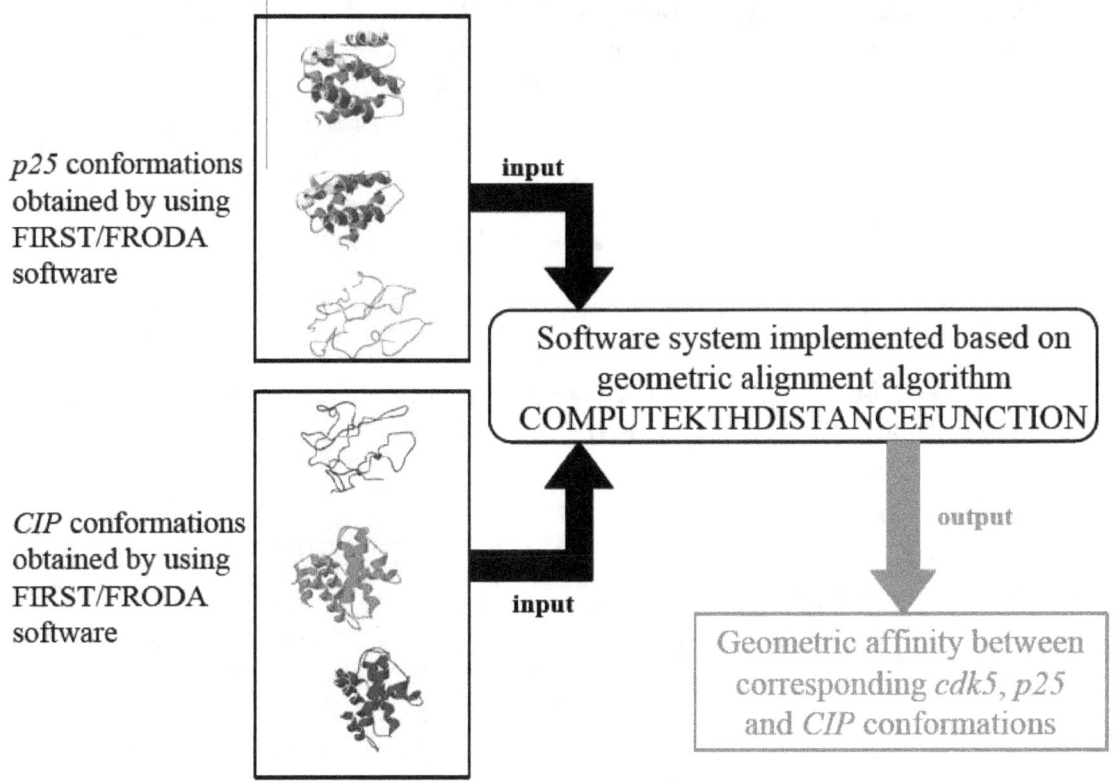

Figure 20. Schematic view of the software system implemented in this work

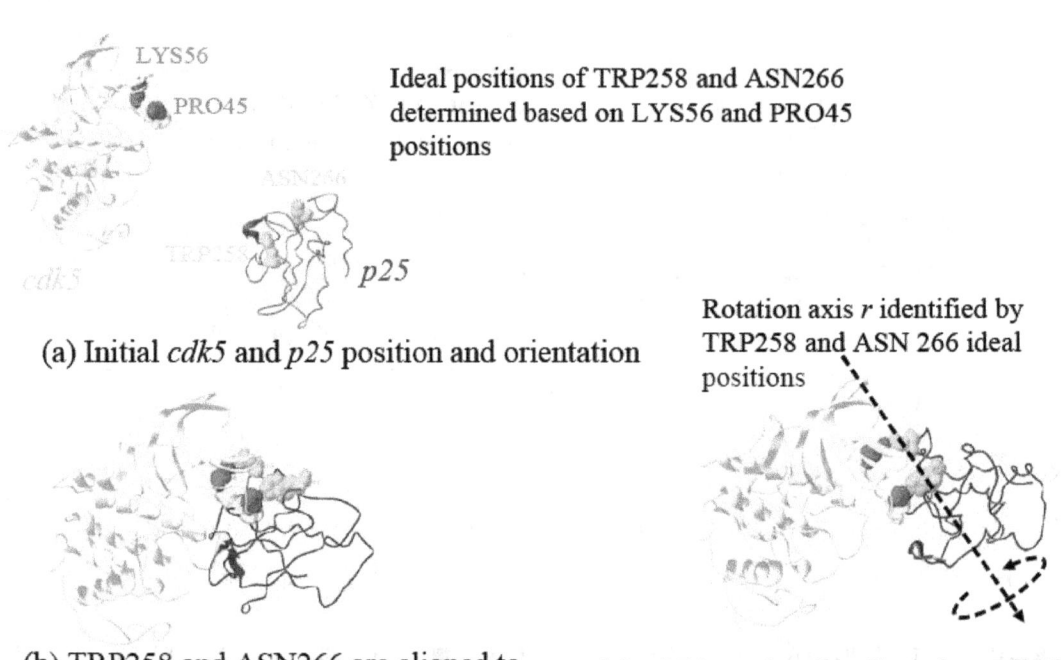

(a) Initial *cdk5* and *p25* position and orientation

Ideal positions of TRP258 and ASN266 determined based on LYS56 and PRO45 positions

Rotation axis *r* identified by TRP258 and ASN 266 ideal positions

(b) TRP258 and ASN266 are aligned to their ideal positions

(c) *p25* is optimally aligned to *cdk5* by rotation around axis *r*

Figure 21. Instance of application of COMPUTEKTHDISTANCEFUNCTION algorithm for a given amino acid pair alignment

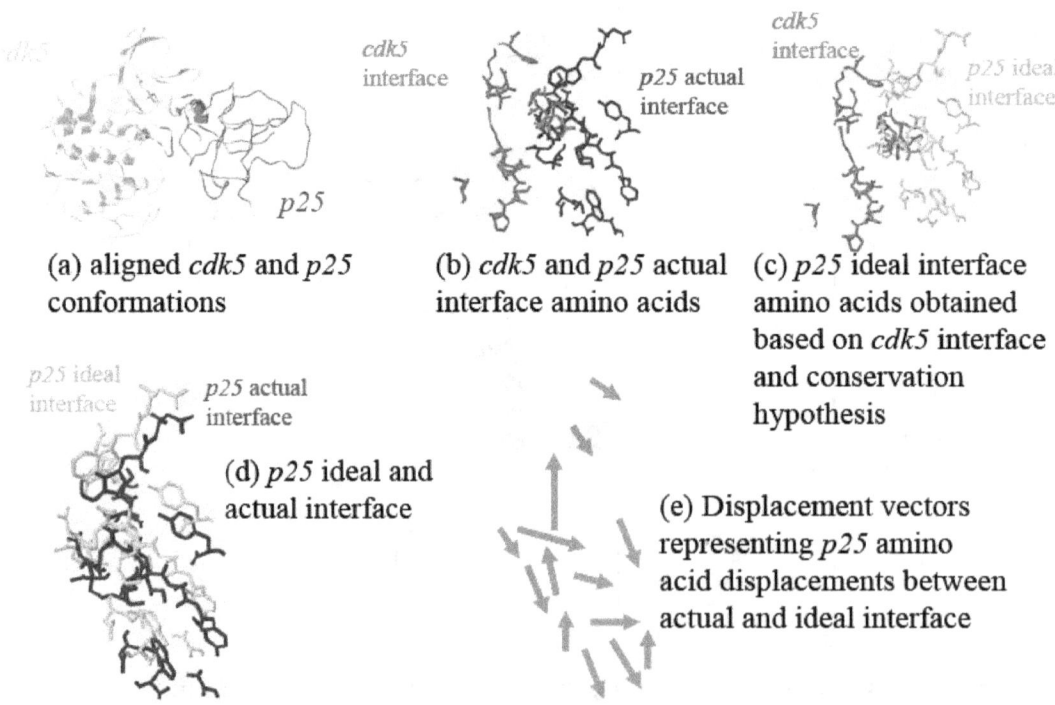

(a) aligned *cdk5* and *p25* conformations

(b) *cdk5* and *p25* actual interface amino acids

(c) *p25* ideal interface amino acids obtained based on *cdk5* interface and conservation hypothesis

(d) *p25* ideal and actual interface

(e) Displacement vectors representing *p25* amino acid displacements between actual and ideal interface

Figure 22. *cdk5* and *p25* are not interacting if the mean norm of displacement vectors shown in (e) exceeds a threshold value

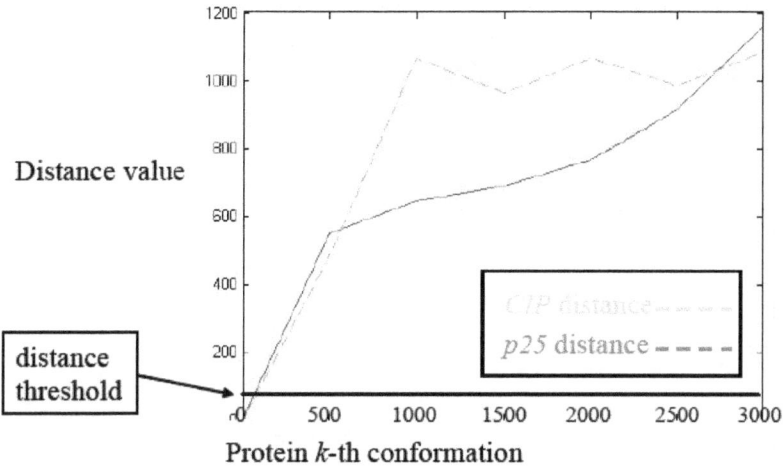

Figure 23. Plot of distance values from Equation (13) vs. *p25* and *CIP* corresponding conformations

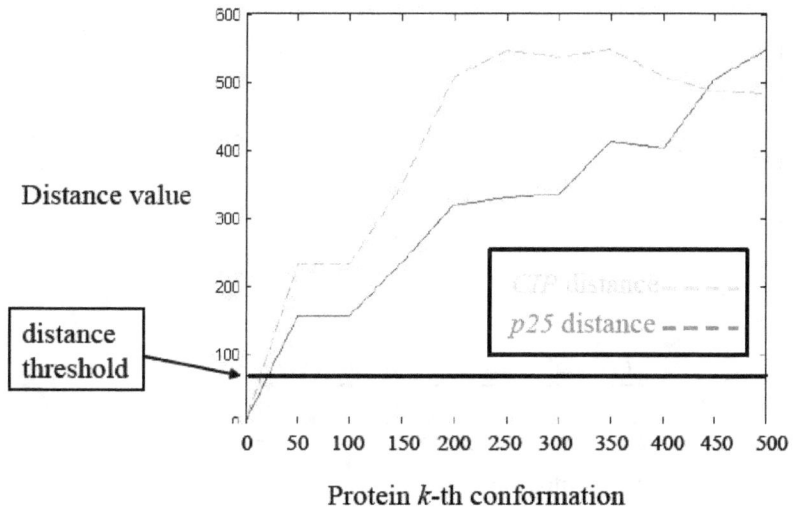

Figure 24. Plot of distance values from Equation (13) vs. *p25* and *CIP* corresponding conformations

51

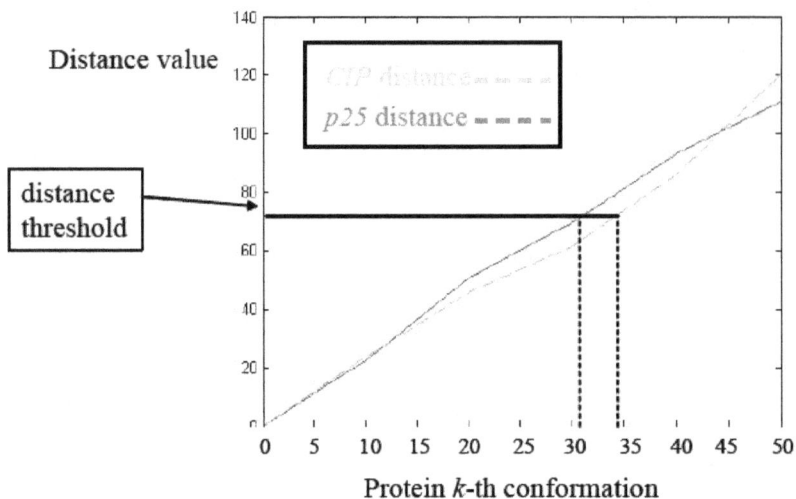

Figure 25. Plot of distance values from Equation (13) vs. *p25* and *CIP* corresponding conformations

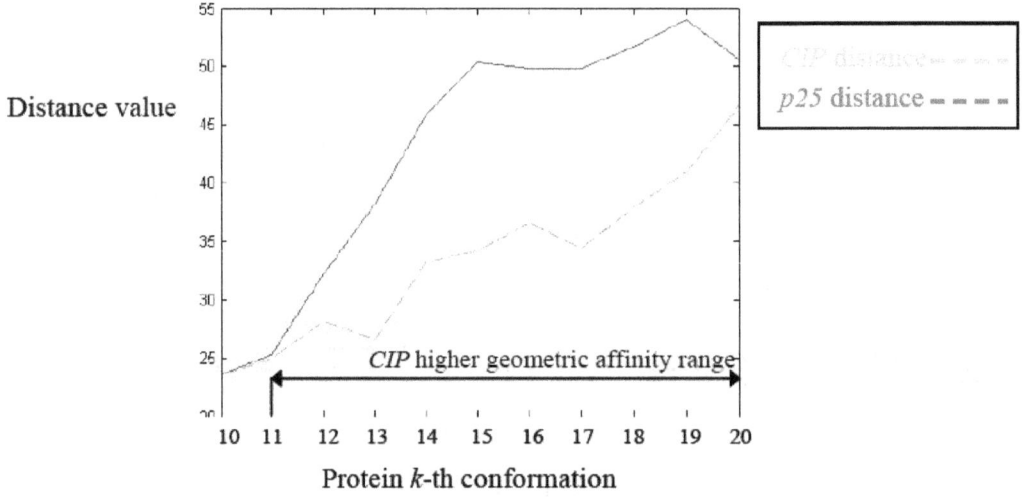

Figure 26. Plot of distance values from Equation (13) vs. *p25* and *CIP* corresponding conformations

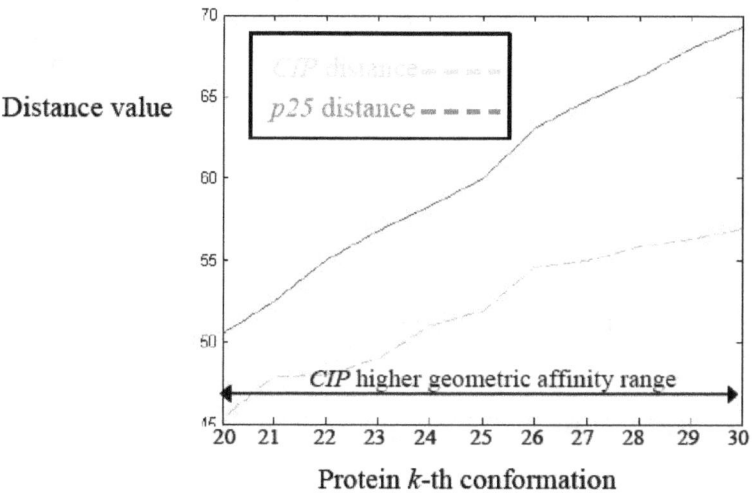

Figure 27. Plot of distance values from Equation (13) vs. *p25* and *CIP* corresponding conformations

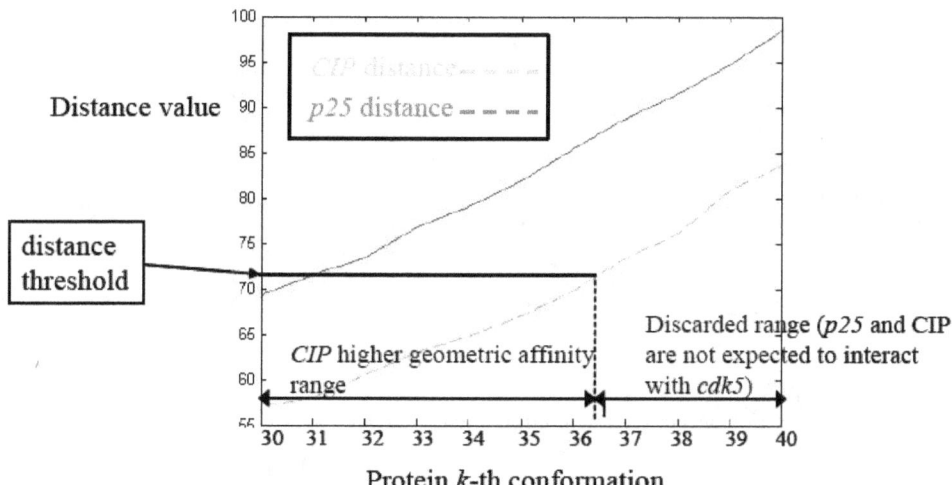

Figure 28. Plot of distance values from Equation (13) vs. *p25* and *CIP* corresponding conformations

53

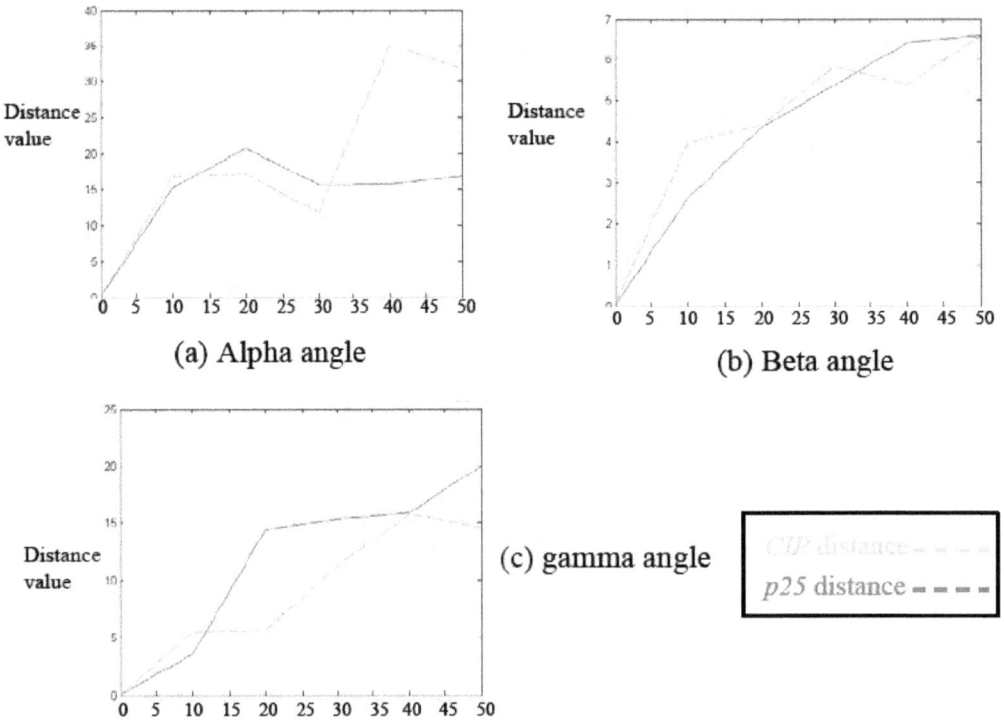

(a) Alpha angle

(b) Beta angle

(c) gamma angle

CIP distance — — — —

p25 distance — — — —

Figure 29. Plot of relative angle values representing interface amino acid relative orientations

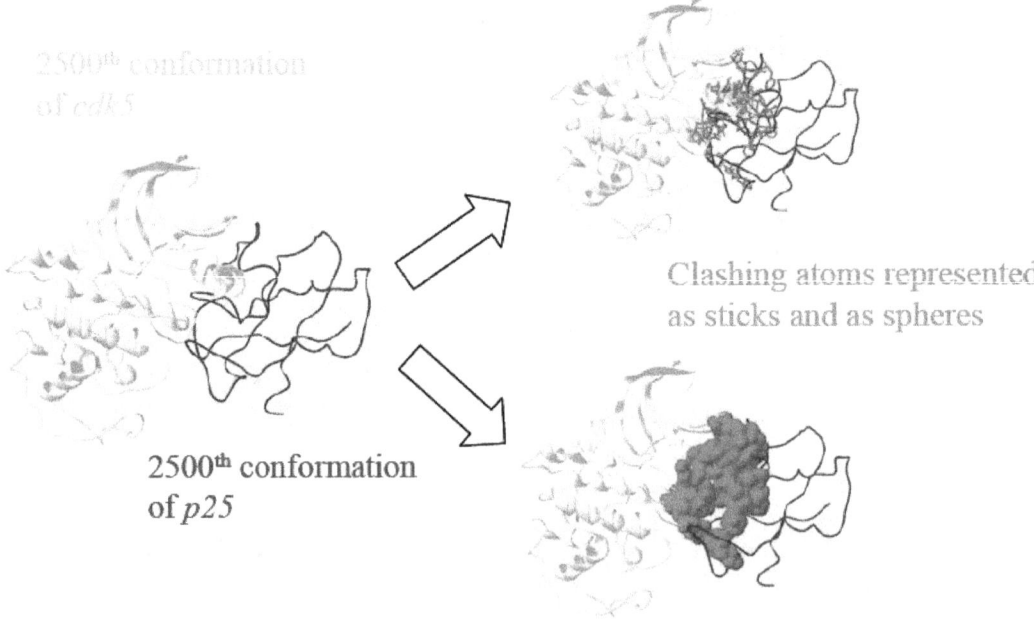

2500th conformation of cdk5

Clashing atoms represented as sticks and as spheres

2500th conformation of p25

Figure 30. Instance of a protein alignment obtained by using our technique that causes a major number of atom clashes

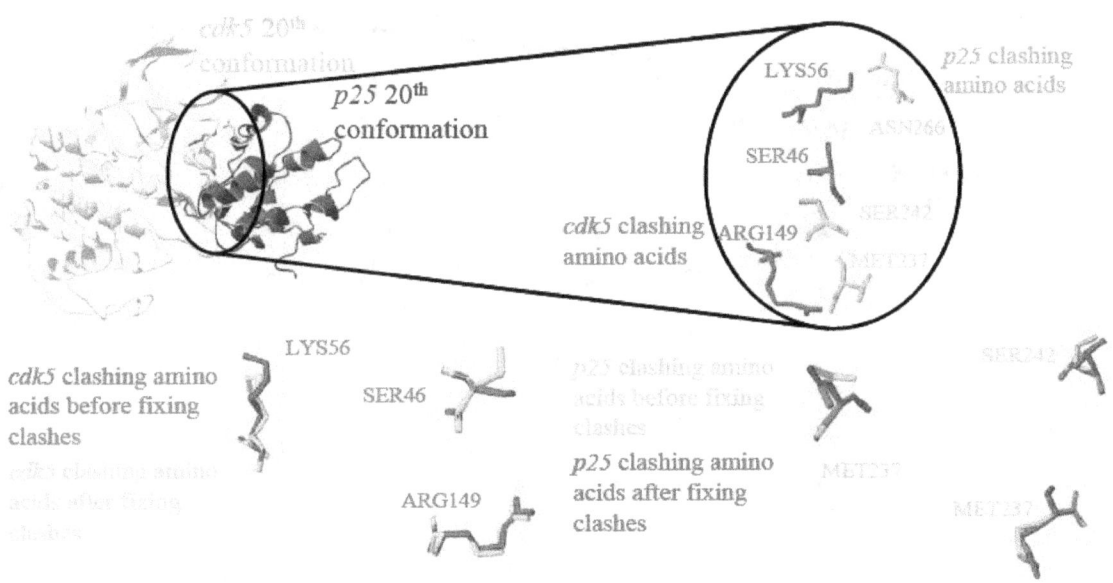

Only little changes in correspondence of amino acid side chains occur

cdk5/p25 distance value yielding geometric affinity before fixing clashes = 52.26
cdk5/p25 distance value yielding geometric affinity before fixing clashes = 54.57

Figure 31. Instance of identification and elimination of clashes for *cdk5/p25* aligned 20ᵗʰ conformations

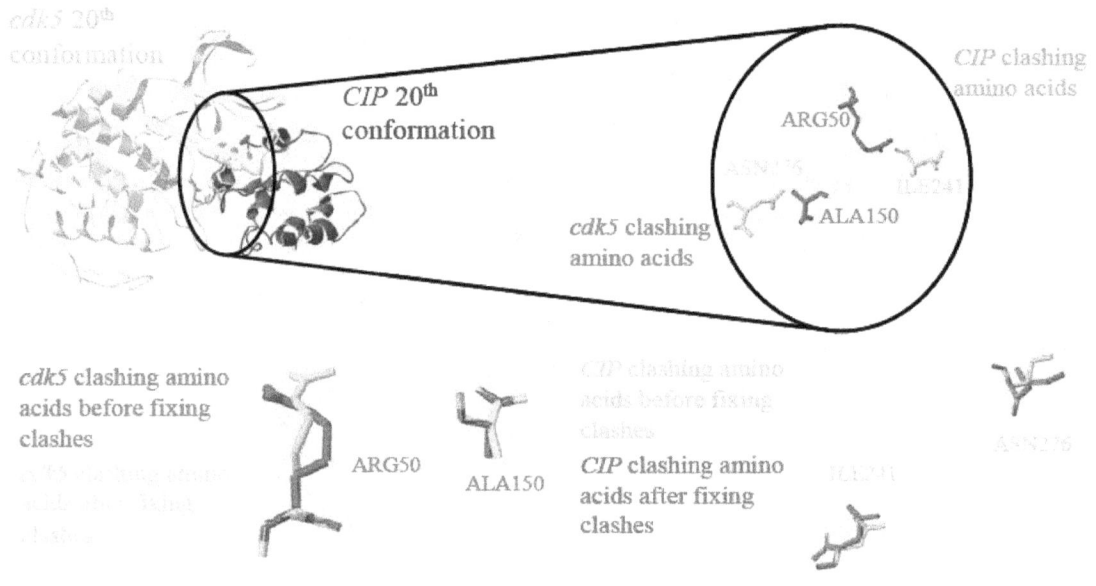

cdk5 clashing amino acids before fixing clashes

CIP clashing amino acids after fixing clashes

ARG50   ALA150

Only little changes in correspondence of amino acid side chains occur

cdk5/CIP distance value yielding geometric affinity before fixing clashes = 47.18
cdk5/CIP distance value yielding geometric affinity before fixing clashes = 48.08

Figure 32. Instance of identification and elimination of clashes for *cdk5/CIP* aligned 20th conformations

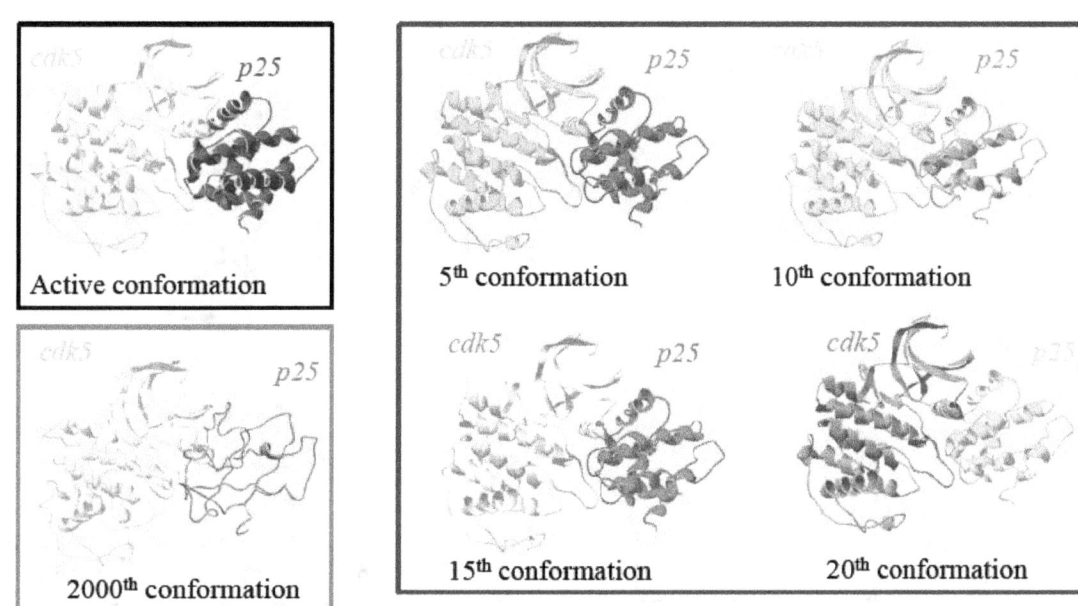

(a) Major clashes are expected for this alignment, which is very different from active complex

(b) No major clashes are expected for these alignments, as they are very similar to active complex

Figure 33. No major clashes are expected for protein alignments very similar to the active complex *cdk5/p25* and vice versa

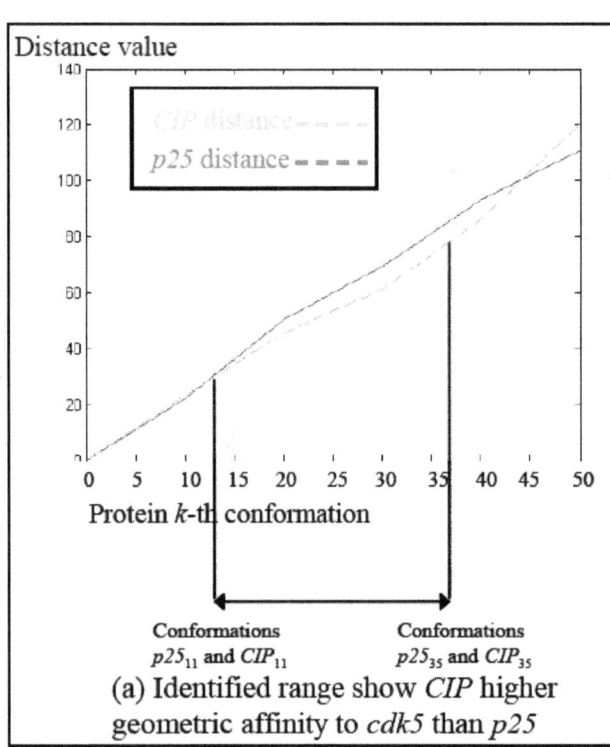

(a) Identified range show *CIP* higher
geometric affinity to *cdk5* than *p25*

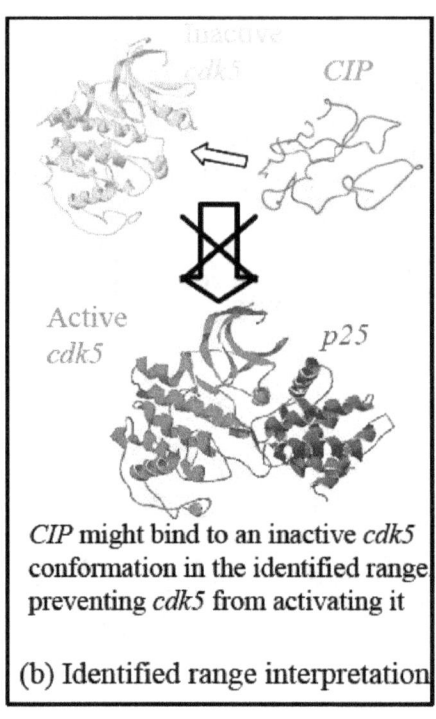

CIP might bind to an inactive *cdk5*
conformation in the identified range
preventing *cdk5* from activating it

(b) Identified range interpretation

Figure 34. Identified range showing *CIP* higher geometric affinity and our interpretation

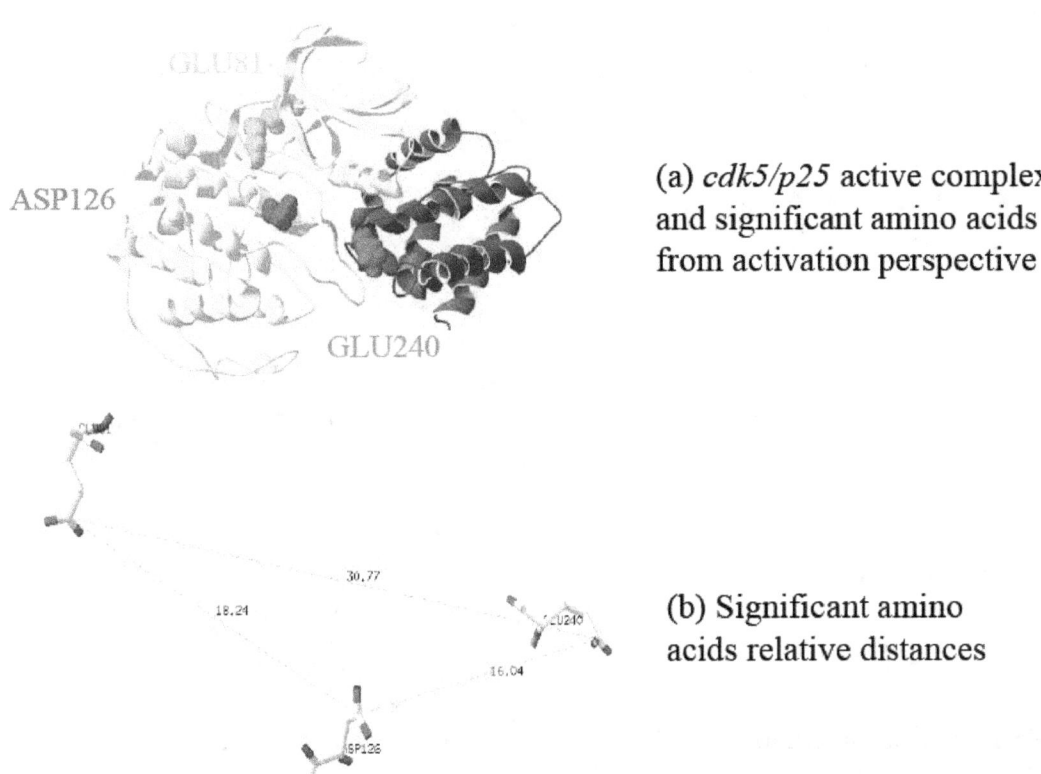

(a) *cdk5/p25* active complex and significant amino acids from activation perspective

(b) Significant amino acids relative distances

Figure 35. Identified amino acids from *cdk5/p25* active complex that are important from activation perspective

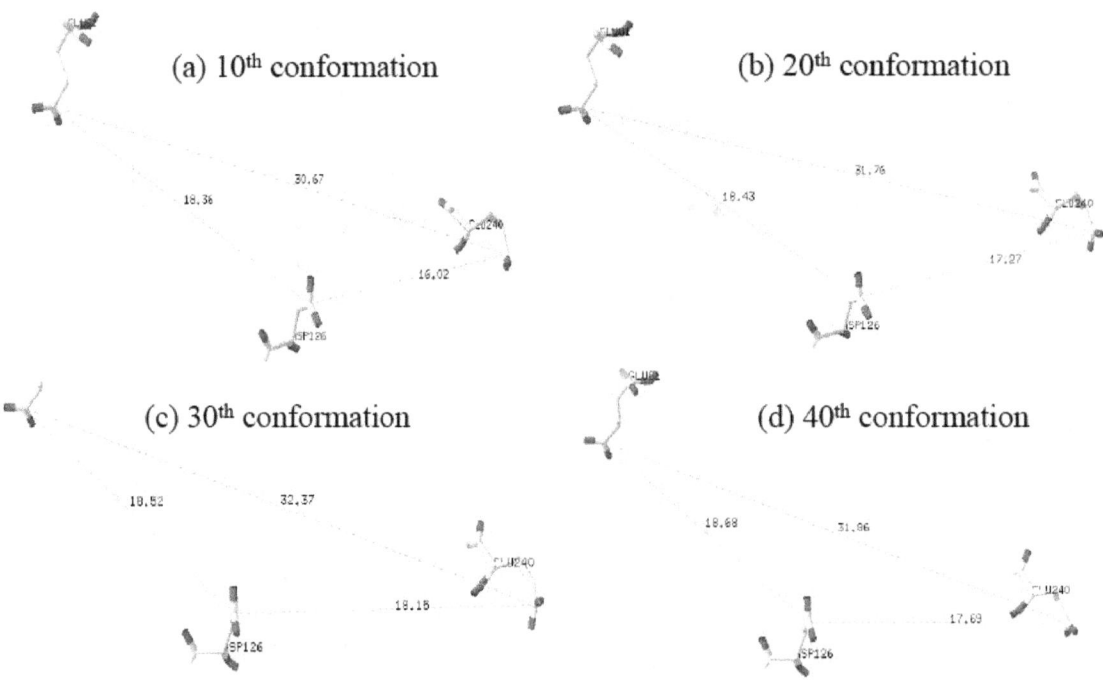

Figure 36. Significant amino acid relative distances from activation perspective for several *cdk5* and *p25* conformations

www.ingramcontent.com/pod-product-compliance
Lightning Source LLC
Chambersburg PA
CBHW081857170526
45167CB00007B/3046